Tantra for the Up and Not Coming Man

And the Woman that Wants to Help Him Keep Going All Night

Kalidasa Brown

Book design by Kalidasa Brown

Yoga Model: Maris Yeager

Liability Disclaimer

This book is presented solely for educational and entertainment purposes only. By reading this book, you assume all risks associated with using the advice given below, with a full understanding that you, solely, are responsible for anything that may occur as a result of putting this information into action in any way, and regardless of your interpretation of the advice.

Terms of Use

Also, there are no resale rights or private label rights granted when purchasing this book. In other words, it's for your own personal use only.

Tantra for the Up and Not Coming Man

And the Woman that Wants to Help Him Keep Going All Night

Contents

Introduction

The average length of intercourse is three to seven minutes, while the "ideal" time is seven to 13 minutes. This is according to various studies and sex therapists.

This is very interesting to me because my lovers have always preferred to have intercourse for a much longer time. Most preferred at least 30 minutes, some much more. It is really nice to be able to accommodate them!

The average numbers could have come from therapists working with men who wanted to increase their ability because they weren't completely satisfying their partners. This book is for all men and women to have greater sexual satisfaction.

I gained the ability to have longer than average intercourse by learning and developing skills. Some came from lovers helping me please them, others I developed on my own. Mainly, everything in this book comes from my personal experience with yoga, tantra and just my love of women.

Restraining an ejaculation is a very difficult thing to do. But, the rewards that come with that ability are obvious. Mainly being able to please a woman like she's never experienced before! That is well worth learning, practicing and perfecting the techniques taught in this book.

While there are many ways to sexually please a woman, most prefer and need a longer time having intercourse to be fully satisfied than most men are capable of. Even if a man is expert at pleasing a woman orally and digitally, I can pretty much guarantee that most women would love having her lover inside her longer.

Of course, the length of time a lovemaking session lasts will and should be much longer than just intercourse. That extra time is essential for women, and it should be a pleasurable time for men as well. Fortunately, some of the practices for restraining ejaculation can be practiced during foreplay. Plus, women can take that time to help teach their man these techniques.

Besides intercourse the couple should have a deep connection with each other, as well as knowing various techniques like how to use your hands and mouth, how to stimulate the g spot, learning your each other's preferences, intercourse techniques and more. This book focuses on extending intercourse time.

Desensitizing

One of the biggest problems men can have during sex is that they just get too stimulated and finish quickly. As harsh as this experience can be for a man, it is actually very easy to help by desensitizing yourself before sex.

There are two very simple ways to do this. First, there are desensitizing creams that work well for some men that are well worth trying. Or, a condom is reliable with the added benefit of protection from disease and pregnancy.

The second way is to desensitize yourself before being with your lover by masturbating. This is also a good time to practice the advanced techniques that this book is mainly about.

The idea is rather simple, though the timing can be difficult. That is, you need to find the ideal time before meeting with your partner to masturbate so you don't get overly stimulated when with her.

All men will lose at least some interest after having sex. A few lucky ones will be able to go again right away while others will need more time to become interested again.

You probably know yourself, at lest somewhat. Young men can often have sex more than once a day and know how often the urge comes upon them. Older or less healthy men may find that once a day is too often and perhaps need several hours to a day or longer to return to readiness.

Whatever is true for you, you will likely need to experiment to find out how long you need to recover. You need to realize though that you will probably need less time to be ready once you are with your lover than it would normally take to be ready again for self stimulation. And, if you are ready quickly after masturbating you are also likely to need to take the edge off just before.

One thing you can count on is that your lover is not likely to care if you need a little more time to recover. The more time you spend with her before intercourse the happier she will be. Of course, there are exceptions, some women don't want to wait all that long, or she might be particularly ready when she sees you, but most will be happy with a little more foreplay.

The key to good foreplay is to love what you are doing. One benefit to her being happy about you needing more time before intercourse is that there is no pressure on her; she won't be thinking you just want to get yours. So, if you masturbated an hour before getting together and you need more time to be ready again, you will be doing the both of you a great favor by learning to enjoy all the amazing things that can be done before you enter her.

Another benefit is that you can take that time to bring her close to orgasm without letting her go over the top. Or better yet, you can keep her at the brink of orgasm for a while. That will insure a massive orgasm and great satisfaction for her while you're in her. The main thing is to get her to a point where she can hardly stand not having you inside her any longer!

With that in mind, it is essential to know your partner, and to know what she needs so you can determine how long before getting together to masturbate your oversensitivity away.

Another thing to think about is that you can masturbate without coming. As hard as it can be, you can get yourself close to orgasm and stop. This can be an especially good technique for men who need more time to be ready again. It is also good for men who aren't sure how much time they may need after masturbating to be stimulated again.

Experimenting without your lover can be important too. That way you can masturbate then wait to see how long until you are able to get yourself erect again. You can bet that you will be able to get there again in that amount of time or less once you are with her!

Another thing you can do is to get your lover involved. Have her take care of you early in whatever way she likes. One of the things that can really satisfy a woman is bringing her lover to orgasm. Or, you might let her watch, some women really like that.

Then, take time to be with each other; talking, cuddling, kissing, massaging and plenty of foreplay for her. Bring her to orgasm without intercourse if she wants. But, plan to have intercourse once you are ready again. This is an especially good thing to do when practicing the techniques you'll soon be learning, that way you can practice with her before intercourse.

Be sure to pay attention to how things work for you, whatever method you use to desensitize. This is one of the easiest ways to be a better lover. And, it can give you space to be with your lover in ways that are satisfying to her.

Introduction to Restraint

There are two methods for restraining an ejaculation. The first, and most common, is the muscular restraint. The second which takes more practice is the energetic restraint. Using both can give you results like you won't believe!

A muscular restraint can release some semen into your ureter which can be drawn up into the bladder with this type of restraint. There isn't usually a lot, but it can be a surprising amount. Ideally, you would stop and restrain before there is any release.

There can also be a loss of drive if there is a seminal release, even just a small amount. Or, your drive and erection can stay strong. It is completely individual.

Usually though, there is at least a little loss of interest for men practicing just the muscular method. A significant loss of interest is more likely if you wait too long to stop and restrain. That is, if you do go too far but are able to fully restrain the ejaculate, you can still lose interest and your erection.

After restraining ejaculation muscularly you can usually see the semen after it is drawn up into your bladder, it comes out when you urinate. There may not be much, but it will probably come out when the urine stream starts. It will look milky, and can be foamy. It will be lighter than your usual ejaculate since it will be diluted with urine.

One thing that can happen to men is that they can have an orgasm without ejaculation, a dry orgasm. That is one reason there can be a loss of desire. But, it is possible to have a dry orgasm with little to no loss of sex drive.

The main factor is general health. The better your health the more likely you will be able to continue with intercourse after restraining an ejaculation, even if you have a dry orgasm.

Also, great health is a very important part of having the ability to stop an ejaculation. Muscular strength is only part of the strength needed for such a difficult practice. Inner strength comes mainly from the adrenal glands.

If you are concerned at all about your optimum sexual health you should really consider looking into adrenal fatigue and how to eliminate it. Even if you enjoy great health, you might like to know how to keep it.

You can learn how to have great health through strengthening the adrenal glands in my book, "Adrenal Fatigue, Get Your Life Back," available on amazon.com.

Energetic ejaculation restraint is a vastly superior method. It may take months or years to master, but it is well worth investing the time.

Even though it may take longer to master than muscular restraint, some results can usually be seen in close to the same amount of time it takes to get results with the muscular technique.

When using both techniques there may still be a slight loss of desire after stopping an ejaculation. This is because a dry orgasm will give you some satisfaction. But, if you stay with your lover and continue intercourse as soon as you can after restraining your desire is likely to flood back in within seconds, a minute or two at most.

The techniques for mastering your energy come from Tantra Yoga, so they are based in yoga. You are not likely to find this information anywhere else, even in tantra books because it is hidden knowledge that is rarely taught.

There are unique breathing techniques, yoga postures, locks (they 'lock' the energy in the body) and even some ethical considerations. You will actually be learning some very advanced techniques.

If practiced regularly, these techniques will have a profound effect on your body, energy and even your life.

Because you will be gaining in ability to influence others, the ethical guidance is essential. The reason is that while your new found abilities can give you short term gratification at the expense of others, the long term damage to you can be astronomical.

Whatever way you might abuse anyone in life you will likely find the opposite effect at a later time. More on this is in the chapter on yoga.

The most important thing is to practice! All the knowledge in the world will do you no good if not put into use. The amount of time spent practicing is totally individual.

Some men, especially if they have great health, will be able to practice more than others since some of the practices use sexual energy. But, no matter what your capacity is, with practice, you will find your sexual abilities increasing over time.

Finally, because these techniques won't absolutely prevent the release of semen every time, these techniques should not be used for birth control. Even if the semen is stopped completely there can still be a small release of fluid containing semen that can result in pregnancy. So, be sure to take your usual precautions.

Muscular Restraint

In this chapter you will learn the basic technique for restraining an ejaculation. This could be one of the most important things you ever learn in regards to sex because it can easily enhance your performance in several ways.

The technique involves squeezing a muscle in the pelvic floor to stop ejaculation, the pubococcygeus muscle, or PC muscle. Both men and women have this muscle. It extends from the pubic bone to the coccyx (tailbone). It is part of the levator ani group of muscles.

You exercise the PC muscle by squeezing your anal area up and in. These contractions will squeeze the ejaculatory duct, and the seminal vesicle as well as the prostate. These are the organ and ducts that carry sperm to the penis.

When the PC muscle is squeezed hard enough and at the right time, it can stop ejaculation. The practice taught in this chapter will strengthen your PC muscle. And, the exercises in the PC muscle exercises section will round out your exercise routine for maximum benefit.

First though, you need to know that orgasm and ejaculation are two separate processes. They usually happen at the same time, and are usually experienced as inseparable. However, you can have an orgasm without ejaculating.

This is sometimes called a dry orgasm where not a single drop of semen is released. As mentioned earlier, you can do this with just a muscular restraint, but you will be much more successful if you learn and practice the energy techniques taught in those chapters.

You need to learn how to separate orgasm and ejaculation. You do this by stimulating yourself until close to orgasm, then stopping. You would also start practicing muscular restraint by squeezing your PC muscle when you stop.

At times you will likely go too far and need to use a really hard squeeze to stop from having an ejaculation and orgasm, that is if you can stop at all at this point in your training.

Also, this practice is a good start for you to find the right time to restrain your ejaculation. There's more information on that coming soon.

Soon after this, you will begin to discover the place where you are starting to orgasm so you know when to withdraw from your partner, or stop masturbating. That may sound like a very tall order, but you can do it.

As you continue to practice you will eventually be able to start to orgasm, catch it, and squeeze your PC muscle to stop before you ejaculate. Finding that place will completely change your experience of sex.

Practicing with yourself is essential, but your partner can help. Tell her what you are doing, and share this material with her. Most likely she'll be happy to help! At any rate you should tell her because some of your lovemaking activities will be different, and could seem strange to her.

One difference is that during intercourse you will need to withdraw when restraining. It is necessary to eliminate all stimulation so there is nothing to tip you over the edge and into ejaculation.

She will need to know that she needs to stop as well when you are restraining. Otherwise, in the heat and passion of the moment, she could easily pull you back in! And, it takes only a little stimulation to tip you into a full release.

As mentioned, when you first start this practice you will need to stop well before you reach the point of no return. Your skill at determining when you are going to pass that point, and when you aren't will developed. Eventually, you will find that there is a magical point between when you start to feel an orgasm coming on, and when ejaculation is certain and no longer controllable.

This gap can be as long as a few seconds, or as short as a small fraction of a second, at least at first. A few lucky men will find the time increasing to where the length of time of intense pleasure and bliss of near orgasm increases. The more you practice, the more likely that will happen to you.

This is a great experience that is really amazing. You will start to experience a different kind of orgasm that can be much more intense than an ejaculatory orgasm; an internal orgasm. You are much more likely to experience an internal orgasm if you do the energy techniques taught later.

At any rate, as your ability to restrain ejaculation increases the time in between an orgasm starting and ejaculation being a surety will become longer and longer. At first though, it will likely be difficult to find exactly where the optimum point to stop and hold is.

At first you will need to stop early, when it is easy to stop yourself from ejaculating, most likely before you experience an orgasm. Gradually go deeper by letting yourself get closer and closer to orgasm before stopping.

You want to find the place where you start to feel an orgasm coming on and then stop and hold. As you practice this, you will be strengthening your PC muscle and opening yourself to the flow of energy that happens with an internal orgasm.

Over time you will get closer and closer to the point of no return. You will probably go past and into a full orgasm with ejaculation at times because experiencing near orgasm without letting go completely is very intense.

Having full stimulation without orgasm can be almost too much to bear, especially if it has been a while since you have ejaculated. At times like this you may let yourself have a full genital orgasm with ejaculation. Sometimes it is just necessary!

Personally, I have gone up to ten months or longer before getting to the point where I had to ejaculate. (It's hard to be sure exactly how long.) But, that's after many years of practice. It's just that at some point it simply becomes impossible to stop yourself!

An important time that you would want to have an ejaculation is if you and your partner are trying to get pregnant. The old sperm should be cleared out because it can become deformed with the DNA even being affected.

Ideally, you would have an ejaculation two days in a row and on the third day try for a child. If she doesn't get pregnant that time, wait till the next time she's ready and do the same thing again.

The main point is to keep practicing until you find the place where you know when you are going to spill over if you go even a fraction of second longer. At that point you may experience an orgasm, or something very similar.

The good news is that you will most likely start to become much better lover during intercourse long before you are able to find that in between point.

One of the most common questions about this practice has to do with sensitive skin on the penis. That can be a real problem for some men. The only thing to do about it is to use plenty of lubrication. Most lotions need to be reapplied, so I recommend light oil or a cream that has oil in it.

Also, the practice will likely help your skin get to where you can masturbate more without problems. You will also get to where you can have intercourse longer without abrasion concerns!

Once you have gotten good at restraining your ejaculation, you will also get to where you can have intercourse longer. Don't be surprised if some of your lovers have sensitive skin and need you to stop because they are rubbed raw! What a great conundrum to find yourself in!

To summarize, the technique is to masturbate until you are close to orgasm, stop and squeeze the PC muscle to keep yourself from ejaculating. There is a whole section on how to strengthen the PC muscle coming up.

Getting Help from a Tantrika

A Tantrika is a woman practitioner of what is sometimes called red tantra. Tantra is a very deep aspect of yoga that has to do with attaining the ultimate state of liberation. Red tantra is a valid branch of tantra that is mostly misunderstood and misused.

In modern red tantra a practitioner, usually a woman or Tantrika, gives a man a genital massage. A lot of Tantrikas will work with both men and women, we'll focus on men.

A good Tantrika will massage your penis until you come close to orgasm and then stop. She is skilled at getting you close without letting you go over the edge.

A very skilled Tantrika can get you to the point where you are on the brink, and hold you there. Or, at least take you to the brink and bring you back several times in a session. You have to expand greatly to be held on the brink!

Red tantra is thought of as Divine work, working with Divine energy. Since all energy is Divine, and sexual energy is a very strong energy, their work is considered more divine in nature.

Because tantra is ideally a Divine practice the sessions are designed to be non-personal. To keep the sexual contact impersonal certain rules are adhered to in a red tantra session. In short, while this practice is sexual, the Tantrika isn't there for a sexual relationship.

To keep this clear both energetically and emotionally, the practitioner takes the role of the "giver" while the recipient is the "receiver." The receiver's job is to stay present with the giver and just receive the pleasure and bliss that comes with this kind of work. The idea is to keep the session impersonal by having it one sided.

Some of the main rules are that there is no intercourse, mouth to mouth kissing, or mouth to genital contact. And, you aren't to reciprocate her loving touch by touching or giving pleasure to her.

These types of sessions can be very intense. The receiver will usually go through a deep inner process that can be about many things. What internal process happens is completely individual, but will usually include dealing with any sexual issues or dysfunction there may be.

Even the most functional man will usually discover something about himself with such a session. It is usually a very emotional experience.

One of the primary purposes of a Red Tantra session is to get through issues that limit an individual from being whole and complete. That is, healing what keeps them from being an autonomous individual, especially in the areas of intimate sexual relationships.

In other words, getting them to a place where they can be fully in a deep and loving relationship, or in whatever type of relationship they wish. That includes getting them to a place where they can be a whole and total individual not in a sexual relationship.

There are also Red Tantra sessions where the woman is the receiver. The method is similar, but different in that women are taken to a very high state of arousal and to orgasm, ultimately a continuous orgasm, through stimulating the G Spot. A good female Red Tantra practitioner will sometimes be willing to teach you how to do this for your lover, possibly even switching roles so you can have practical experience as the giver with her as the receiver.

There is a lot more to Red Tantra than mentioned here, that's for another book. What ultimately happens depends on both the giver and the receiver, and where they are in their process and knowledge.

Most men will likely elect for practicing with themselves. For one thing, Red Tantra sessions and workshops are expensive.

For another, a man is more likely to spend more time masturbating even if he gets a session from time to time. And, it is generally better for a man to start practicing restraint alone, even if he decides to eventually get sessions.

Learning more about red tantra is another way to increase your ability as a lover. And, learning with your lover is a great way to increase the joy of sex with her as well as deepening your relationship.

There are a fair number of tantra teachers around these days. Workshops are a great way to learn. And, you may be able to learn from books. I will likely write some myself, and am happy to give private sessions, especially to couples.

PC Muscle Exercises

There are several benefits to exercising your PC muscle. Mainly of course is giving you the ability to control ejaculation.

Squeezing the PC muscle also reduces the stimulation to orgasm. It also helps desensitize the urge to orgasm. At the very least, it can dampen the urge.

Another is that it helps your prostate health by massaging it. The practice keeps the blood flow strong and helps push out toxins. It can even help prevent or reduce BPH, a swollen prostate which can help alleviate problems urinating.

There are other sexual benefits as well. It can make your penis stronger and more muscular looking. Women aren't generally visually oriented when it comes to sex, but they often do appreciate a nice looking penis.

Another big sexual benefit is that you will be able to pulse your penis inside her. This gives a completely different sensation that many women really like. Some women's anatomy is such that these pulses can stimulate her G spot, which she will *really* love.

Another benefit is that you can do these exercises with your lover. The PC exercise is the same as Kegel exercises that many women learned to do when young. Mostly they are taught so they can control urine leaks.

Another effect on women who do Kegel exercises that you will love is that they develop a tighter vagina, which is great on its own. But, she will also be able to give your penis an amazing squeeze during intercourse. There is nothing like having a lover who can squeeze you while you move in and out of her!

Also, both men and women will usually have stronger orgasms if they have strong PC muscles. Even the ejaculate will be more forceful (when you have one) which is great for both of you.

You can exercise together most anytime. Reminding each other to practice can even be another way to bond. You could practice together while in the car, watching TV, at the movies or while taking a stroll, just about any time you can think of.

PC exercises are difficult to do when walking, especially at first. That gets easier once the PC gets some strength. And, it is mostly impossible to practice when running.

A really great time to do PC exercises together is when you are inside her. In fact, there is a tantra technique in which you hold still while she squeezes and you flex inside her. That can be a great experience once your rhythm together develops.

Another benefit for the both of you is that one of the exercises can make you bigger! Don't do just that one though; you really need to practice them all to get a well-rounded workout.

You can do these exercises, except the one that makes you bigger, in any position; sitting, lying down or even while standing in line.

The only limit is while you are eating. It just doesn't work very well because digestion takes the majority of your blood flow. Generally, you should wait at least 30 minutes after eating just to make sure you get the full benefit.

The basic exercise is to simply contract and release your genital/anal area.

How do you know if you have the right muscle? Simple, stop your urine flow. The muscle you squeeze to stop your flow is the PC muscle.

It is important to warm up before you start exercising the PC. Yes, it is like exercising any other muscle that needs to be warmed up before strenuous exercise.

The great thing is that the basic exercise is the same whether you are exercising or warming up; it's just a matter of intensity. To warm up you simply contract the PC for about two seconds, then completely relax for a couple of seconds. Do three sets of 12 to 15 repetitions with a 15 second rest between sets. Start easy and squeeze harder with each set so you are squeezing as hard as you can with the last set.

Once you have warmed up you can do the exercises as much as you like, the more the better. You should strive to do a lot, even a thousand or more a day after building up from two or three hundred a day.

One thing to watch out for is tightening other muscles. You need to keep all other muscles relaxed when working your PC. The most common muscles that need to be kept relaxed are the thighs, abdominals and the buttocks. Keeping these areas relaxed insures that the PC muscle is well targeted for full benefit.

Another thing to watch out for, especially when you first start out, is that you might actually get sore. It isn't common to get really sore, though it is possible that you'll notice something. The cure is a gentle PC workout.

Sore muscles are caused by a natural buildup of a toxin called lactic acid which is a byproduct of muscle use. Lactic acid often builds up in muscles that aren't used to working a lot. Exercising the area lightly helps the lymph system move the lactic acid out resulting in the soreness going away.

You will be able to exercise more once you do a light PC workout and the soreness leaves. However, if the soreness doesn't leave, or if the muscles are left feeling tight or very tired then you can either have a light workout day, or skip the day. After a short time the area won't generally get sore any more, just like other muscles you might exercise.

That all being said, here are the exercises:

Standard Contractions

This is the standard contractions you've already learned. With each contraction tighten up fully, and then relax completely. Eventually you'll work up to doing hundreds. You can work up to a thousand a day for the days you are doing just this particular workout.

Work in sets of 25 once you have warmed up. Take a break of about a minute between each set. If you can do ten sets, that's great, especially to begin with. If you work up to forty sets then you will have done a thousand standard contractions!

You do not have to do them all at one time. You can spread out your contractions throughout the day. Just be sure to warm up if it's been awhile since your last workout.

Flutters

PC Flutters are like standard contractions, except you contract and release quickly without contracting as strongly as you can.

Flutters are done for endurance. You want to see how long you can keep going. Try to do the flutter exercise for one minute, and then rest for one to three minutes. Repeat at least five times. Do more if you like, but while this exercise is important, it isn't the most important one.

Flex and Hold

The Flex and Hold workout is more advanced, and the most important exercise. It should be done most every day since it is what you are going to be doing to stop ejaculations. However, it is best to start with the first two PC exercises for two to five days before doing a lot of this one.

The exercise is to simply squeeze and hold the PC tightly for a count of ten to start. Start with three to four times a day with at least a minute relaxation in between.

You really need to build up on this one. Work towards holding for a max of two minutes. That is generally the longest you will need to hold to restrain an ejaculation, though you will generally only need to hold for a minute or less to restrain most ejaculations.

You also want to work up to doing this several times a day. How many depends on how many times you need to hold back an ejaculation during sex. That can be anywhere from just a few to a hundred or more. Of course, having sex is a good way to do this PC exercise!

Intensity Increases

This is another more advanced exercise for the PC. You start with a light contraction of the PC holding for three or four seconds. Then, without releasing, squeeze more, about half strength and hold for three or four seconds. Finally squeezing as hard as you can for three or four seconds.

Release in opposite order by relaxing a little and pause, then relax to a light squeeze, and finally relax all the way. Relax completely for 30 seconds and do another set.

Work up to ten or more sets a day using this exercise as an add-on exercise. Keep doing the long hold PC exercise on a regular basis; just do this one every three or four days, or as a way to vary your routine.

Find the Beat

This PC exercise can be fun, though the concentration required can be difficult. One way you can do this is to do the contractions in time to the beat of music you are listening to.

You can get imaginative with this practice. For example, you can squeeze and hold till a light changes. Or, hold for as long as it takes an attractive woman you notice to cross the street. Find something that interests you as a way to make the exercise more entertaining.

The Hanging Cloth

This is the one that can make bigger!

Once you've developed some strength with the above exercises you can try this advanced weight lifting PC exercise. At first, use a washcloth as a weight to lift with your erect penis.

Stand and drape the cloth over your erect penis, cover the entire penis, and lift the cloth by squeezing your PC muscle. Lift and lower several times.

How many repetitions depends on how much you have already exercised your PC muscle, and how much strength you have developed. In general, do the previous exercises at least two weeks before weight lifting.

Three sets of three is a good place to start with weight lifting. Build up over time to as many as feels comfortable. Five sets of five is a good average for most men.

Eventually, you can start to wet the cloth for more weight. Wring it out well at first, and keep it dripping wet once you've developed more strength. Increase to a hand towel, and then if you get really strong you can use a bath towel. Use your best judgment and work with what you can actually lift.

Work this exercise into your regular routine. One way to do this is to do a few after a shower. And, a hot shower is a great warm up so you don't strain the PC muscle.

After a while your lover will be amazed at the sensations you can give her by squeezing your PC muscle while inside her. Give her something to brag to her friends about!

Growing bigger from this exercise comes from the gentle pressure of the cloth on your penis which will stimulate growth. Covering it completely helps facilitate the stimulation that causes the tissue to respond by growing.

Those are the PC muscle exercises. Practice the squeeze and hold the most, and mix in the others as you are able. You should start to see results fairly quickly, especially when you do the weight lifting since your strength will obviously increase.

You can do your PC exercises pretty much anytime while doing most anything, as long as it isn't going to distract you. Get in the habit of daily exercise as soon as you can. Remember, the more you exercise, the better you will be able to please your lover!

If you practice these exercises regularly you will find it almost easy to restrain an ejaculation. However, there is always a point where you won't be able to stop no matter how strong you are. The energetic method takes up where the strength method leaves off.

Note:
One technique that is always mentioned by other people teaching how to stop ejaculation is the

mechanical hold. This simple technique can be done by you or your lover. However, it isn't nearly as powerful as having a strong PC muscle and squeezing before you have no choice but to ejaculate.

What you do is use your fingers to squeeze the underside base of your penis to keep from ejaculating.

Another technique that is taught is to squeeze where the skin joins the tip of the penis. Try them both to find the one that works best for you.

This may be a good technique for some men, however I have never heard from men I taught that it works that well. It is well worth trying, especially at first before you have developed PC muscle strength through exercise.

Introduction to Energetic Restraint

The body is full of energy. According to yoga physiology it circulates through 880,000 energy channels and seven primary energy centers (chakras).

This energy is what keeps the body going. Good health and vitality are present when the energy flows freely, while blockages cause illness and lassitude.

There are amazing things that can be done with this energy. All it takes is knowledge of how to make it work for you, and practice from that knowledge.

The techniques presented here are specifically for restraining ejaculation, but the energy developed can be used in other ways as well. For example, pleasing your lover sexually, or even attracting a lover.

The techniques taught in the next chapters can make you a very potent person in life as well as sexually. There is a lot of willpower used to restrain an ejaculation. This willpower will translate into greater willpower in your life. The techniques presented here for learning how to do this are more powerful than just about anything you will ever learn.

There are both active and sitting techniques involved in developing these abilities. The active ones are a set of yoga postures combined with breathing techniques and energy locks to drive your energy up. This will all be explained in detail.

These yogic techniques, while ancient, are not usually taught and so are very difficult to find. I present information here that comes from over 30 years of deep meditation and study.

The sitting meditation is also ancient, but is fairly easy to find in contemporary books. In fact, it is the basis of qigong, literally energy cultivation. It is something you can do most any time you have a minute or two, so it is good for busy people. It also comes from what I have learned and practiced most of my adult life.

As you learn these techniques you may have questions. I have tried to include everything you need to learn in order to practice restraining an ejaculation, but I am only human.

Since the techniques are universal, a few people may have questions that are not necessarily related. You can contact me, and I'll try to answer any questions you may have. They may be answered at kalidasa.com

The two techniques can be practiced concurrently, which is ideal. Depending on your disposition you may find one more preferable to practice than the other. That is fine, but you should at least try to practice both as they are synergistic. That is, the effects of both together are much greater than the sum of the parts.

Men who practice both the energetic and energy methods of restraint are likely to find huge shifts happening to them. The same is true for women. But, while there are similarities, the specifics are for another book. In other words, women can practice these techniques to increase their sexual pleasure as well as to effect changes in their lives.

A big shift that may happen for a few men is that they may find themselves using just the energy method to restrain ejaculations. That is ultimately superior to the muscular method. However, that path is long requiring a lot of guidance, and usually, years of practice.

Consequently, it is best to work with both the muscular and energetic techniques together. After a while you may start to experience the deeper attributes that are related to the energy method.

Energy Circulation Technique

Energy Circulation techniques have been around for millennia. They have been taught to and used by kings and monks alike. They have been passed down as well as developed independently by just about every long lasting civilization the world has had. The form may vary, but they are fundamentally the same.

The basic idea is to cause sexual energy to move up. Normally, sexual energy moves up from the time we are born until puberty when the energy starts on its downward path. That manifests mainly as ejaculation and menstruation.

Changing that path is a herculean task that usually can be accomplished for only short periods of time. For example, pulling the energy up rather than having it move down in an ejaculation.

The Energy Circulation technique helps by circulating the energy up the back and down the front. This keeps both upward and downward flow in harmony. But, at least some of the time is spent moving the energy up which increases willpower and abilities.

When doing the technique you will be dealing with two of the main energy channels in the body. Both start at the perineum, the area between the genitals and anus. In yogic physiology that is the root chakra, or root energy center.

One energy channel runs from the perineum up the back, to the crown of the head, then down through the brain to the hard palate at the roof of the mouth. The other runs from the perineum up the front of the body to the tip of the tongue.

To circulate the energy you need to connect the two channels by lightly touching your tongue to the roof of the mouth. The ideal position is with the tongue touching the hard palate just before it ends at the soft palate at the back of the mouth.

You can find this by tracing your tongue back along the hard palate until you reach the soft palate. Use some pressure so you can feel where the palate changes. The ideal place to hold your tongue is at the hard ridge just before the soft palate.

For some people that point can be hard to reach with the tongue. Holding the tongue there while focusing on circulating the energy can be even harder. While that is the ideal place to hold the tongue, anywhere else on the hard palate between that ridge and the back of the front teeth will work.

To be clear, anywhere in the center of the hard palate between just behind the front teeth to the end of the hard palate will work. It is good to stretch yourself somewhat by reaching your tongue back a little further than is perfectly comfortable for the best results since the further back the more powerful. Also, by doing that you will stretch your tongue so you can move your tongue further back over time.

Energy follows attention. That is, your energy will go wherever you put your attention. You have likely experienced this when someone who is interested in you puts their attention on you. You can feel their energy, sometimes before you even notice they are looking at you.

Moving the energy in your body follows the same principle. You put your attention on where you want your energy to be, and it will go there.

The direction you want the energy to flow in the energy circulation technique starts at the perineum moving up to the back of your head to the crown. From there you would bring your attention and energy straight down to the point of contact between your hard palate and tongue.

Keep your attention on the point of contact between your tongue and the hard palate for a few breaths. Next, you'll bring your attention and energy down the front of your body and back to the perineum.

The speed of the energy movement depends on your disposition, and what is happening with your energy in the moment. So, there is a faster and a slower technique. Each has a different breathing technique as well.

The faster technique is to **bring your energy up the spine to the crown of your head with a long slow inhale, then taking it to the palate and tongue connection during part of the exhale. Hold at the tongue/palate connection for three to five breaths. Follow that with a long slow exhale as you bring the energy down the front and to the perineum again for the next inhale to continue the circulation.**

The slow technique is to bring the energy up the spine in stages. Use a long slow inhale to bring the energy up as far as it wants to go, usually around the small of the back.

Continue to bring the energy up to different areas of your back with each inhale. The second stopping point might be somewhere between your shoulder blades. Your third inhale might bring it up to the back of your neck. Then use another breath to bring it to the back of your head, then the crown of your head with another inhale.

You could then have the energy in your brain for two or three breaths. Then you would exhale to bring the energy and your attention to the point where the tongue and palate contact and hold there for several breaths, as long as three minutes or so. In fact, three minutes is the ideal time to keep your attention at that point.

Afterward, continue the slow method by bringing the energy down the front in a similar way. The first exhale could bring it to your throat or chest area. The diaphragm, belly and genitals are other good pausing points. Keep your attention on the pause point as you take your next slow deep inhale before moving the energy down to the next point as you exhale.

The suggested pause points are just suggestions. Your energy will find the ideal place to pause. All you have to do is let go and allow whatever is perfect for you in the moment to happen.

Generally, the first technique is what most people will find works best. Try the slow method out a few times though, it can be very peaceful. A good time to do that one is when you are going to sleep because it can help you fall asleep. You won't be able to finish as described below, but that is ok, sleep is a good finish, at least some of the time.

Continue to circulate the energy in this way, however fast you go, until you are ready to finish. Ideally, you will a set length of time to practice. Setting a timer is best, but be sure to allow for a little time to finish because the ending is very important.

On the final circuit, as you exhale the energy down the front, stop the energy in your belly starting at a point just below your belly button. Focus your attention there for at least 30 seconds as you do a normal to slightly deep diaphragmatic breath. Feel the energy fill your belly as you exhale into the area. This is where you will store your energy at the end of your practice.

Diaphragmatic breathing is breathing in the belly only without the chest rising or falling at all. You can practice with one hand on your belly and one on your chest so you know where the breath is going until you get the hang of it.

If you have trouble with diaphragmatic breathing a good way to practice is while lying on your back, it is usually easier to do in that position. Breathing in through the nose and out through the mouth is ideal. Also, use controlee with breathing techniques for maximum benefit.

Storing the energy in the belly is important because it is from there that the energy, including the ejaculatory energy, is drawn up from the genitals. There's more information on this later in the discussion on the locks.

After a few months practice you can think about storing the energy in your heart area instead. That is the entire chest area starting at the solar plexus.

The reason this is a good area to store the energy is that it has to do with Divine love. As you practice these energy techniques you will naturally become a more caring person with a greater ability to be in deep contact with others, especially your lover. It's completely up to you if and when you start this storage practice.

The above are the general instructions for Energy Circulation. Not everyone will be able to just start experiencing the energy circulation, so here are some techniques for developing the ability to build and experience the energy more deeply.

Intensifying Energy Circulation

Experiencing the energy while practicing Energy Circulation can be elusive when you first start.

The main thing to remember is that energy follows attention. Your energy will always go wherever you put your attention.

This is true in life as well as in the Energy Circulation technique. That is why this technique is so powerful; it trains you to master your energy.

For example, if you keep your attention on finding a loving partner to be with, you are more likely to draw her to you. You know she's out there because you put your attention on her, even if you haven't met her yet. And, on some level, she feels that attention and gets your energy. And, because of your previous attention, she's sure to feel something when you meet.

The same is true for pleasuring your partner. Just the fact that you bought this book and are reading it will already give you more energy to be attentive to your partner's sexual needs and desires.

Practicing these techniques will increase that even more, not just because you are learning and practicing something that will give you an amazing ability, but because your attention is on *her* and *her* pleasure.

Even if you are studying this material to find and greatly please more women, you are putting your attention and therefore your energy towards those women. On some level they experience this, and so, they are more likely to show up and want to be with you.

In the same way, when you put your attention on your spine and imagine the energy flowing as your attention moves up your spine you are actually moving the energy whether you experience it or not. Just by continuing to practice circulating your energy by imagining the energy flow you are in fact moving and therefore circulating your energy.

Eventually, you will experience the energy as you move your attention through your body. This is true in life as well! You will gain the ability to feel, see or sense energy around you.

You will also start knowing where your partner is putting her attention because of the energy shift. You will instantly know what she wants and needs in your lovemaking!

If you are single, you will gain the ability to notice others energy and attention when you are open to meeting someone special. You will become able to direct your energy towards someone you are interested in, which can be very attractive to them if done right. And, it will become much easier to know when someone is interested in you (or not, so you can move on).

How long it takes to start seeing results is very individual. It all depends on how much time you spend circulating your energy, and how regular your practice is. Thirty minutes a day is an ideal time, though some people will be interested in doing more or less. Consistency is the key.

Many people will start to notice changes in themselves within a month or two especially if they do a longer practice. Others may take more time. The general guideline is to give it a year and a quarter of regular practice before evaluating how something like this is affecting you.

Another way to increase the energy flow and your experience of it is to learn directly from someone by induction. Being in the presence of a master of this technique while they are doing it can transfer that energy and the feel for it, to you in a deep way.

A good way to find someone is to take qigong classes from a qigong master. Ask if they know this particular Energy Circulation technique. Describe it to them, they will likely know it. Then, get them to do it in your presence while you practice as well.

One off the most powerful ways you can kick off this energy for yourself is by doing one of the PC muscle exercise. This is similar to what is taught in the advanced yoga techniques taught in the next chapters.

Squeezing your PC muscle is a great way to kick the energy up your spine in a way that you can have a clear experience of it. The technique is to squeeze your PC muscle as you inhale the energy up your spine. Keep squeezing throughout the inhale. Relax the PC muscle when the energy reaches the crown of the head, and continue circulating the energy as usual.

Once the energy is back at the perineum, you would do another PC squeeze to bring the energy up again. Continue with the energy circulating technique using a PC contraction each time you inhale to help the energy up your spine.

It isn't necessary to do the practice with PC squeezes all time, but it is a good practice that can really help you to have a good experience of the energy when you are first starting out. It is also a good way to practice your PC exercises as well as getting you prepared for the energetic restraint technique.

Whatever your experience of the energy flow is, you will get more and more of a sense of it as you continue practicing. Eventually, you will start to notice unexpected changes in your body, health and abilities. I really can't express fully how powerful this technique is, but if you practice diligently, you will experience changes.

Introduction to Energy Restraint

The following sections contain some of the most power techniques you will ever find for stopping an ejaculation. It contains information that you are not likely to find anywhere else. You can probably find pieces of it from various sources, but I have never seen it in this complete form.

It is also one of the most powerful energy boosting techniques you will ever find. If you are generally healthy then you will find your energy increasing within just a few days or weeks of practice, maybe even after your first time practicing just the locks.

When any animal has sex, the energy moves downward and out of the body. Stopping an ejaculation has the general effect of moving that energy upward. I say "general" because there is always some downward movement of energy that naturally happens with any sexual activity.

Causing sexual energy to move upward is actually fairly easy for women when it comes to sex, but almost impossible for men. All most women need is to be told to pull their orgasm up their spine, or to pull their energy up their spine when they have an orgasm.

This causes them to have a full body orgasm. A lot of women have this type of orgasm already, especially if they build up to orgasm, or if they tend to have bigger and bigger ones during sex.

For a man to experience a full body orgasm they *have* to have an internal orgasm without ejaculation. For that to happen, he needs to have at least one of the three locks occur.

There are three locks that can happen. They **lock** the energy in the body so it can't escape in the downward flow that accompanies ejaculation. Their general function is to force the energy to move up.

Force is a bit of a strong word to use here because the energy is more driven up. And, it is done in a different way than what is usually thought of when words like "force," or "driven" are used.

It is more of a Divine experience that is difficult to explain. This isn't the place to discuss that in detail, just understand that there is something significantly different than what you may normally think in this context.

When an internal orgasm happens for a man it usually happens as a full body orgasm with little or no loss of desire to continue having intercourse. You will have to stop to allow that deep orgasm happen while you restrain the ejaculation, but you will probably be able to continue right after.

One of the side benefits to this is that when you have a full body upward flow orgasm like this, your lover will almost always have the same experience, at least in female terms since women's orgasms are significantly different from a man's.

Women are much more likely to have the capacity to have a full body orgasm like that over and over again. They naturally tend to be multiply orgasmic. Having an orgasm that is induced by her lover's internal orgasm can be very special and different for her.

In other words, the pleasure you give her during intercourse will be more than she has likely ever experienced with any man before, or than she is likely to experience in the future. And, having more intercourse time is one of the ways she is likely to have multiple orgasms that build in intensity to a massive female type of full body orgasm.

Women who don't have full body orgasms, or who are not multiply orgasmic can usually be brought to that kind of experience with a red tantra practitioner who is expert at stimulating the G spot, or with a lover who is trained in those techniques. Red tantra for women is for another book, but your lovemaking skills can definitely make the difference for her.

The locks that are taught here are sometimes presented in yoga classes. Having the locks occur spontaneously isn't so common though. How to use the breath to bring about the locks spontaneously is one of the keys to unlocking upward flow.

The short yoga class presented in this book can be done in as little as 20 minutes or so. Or, a more intense practice can be done that could take up to 45 minutes or more.

This yoga class is designed to move the energy up from the perineum to the crown of the head, moving through each of the seven energy centers. That is, from the first to the seventh chakra.

The final goal is to be able to use a breathing technique when you restrain ejaculation that will bring on the locks and drive the energy up into a full body orgasm without ejaculation. That type of orgasm will be very different from what you are used to. It will course through you like an electric shock that sends waves of pleasure through your body.

This is both more satisfying and less satisfying than a normal orgasm. For me, in a lovemaking session like that, I get driven to have more and more intercourse with my lover. As long as I don't ejaculate even a drop it's like I just can't stop!

The ultimate satisfaction of an ejaculation is denied with more and more of a drive to have it. It is both nerve wracking and amazingly blissful at the same time. It's as if something else takes over that I am at the mercy of.

Most of my lovers haven't had the capacity to continue having intercourse with me for nearly as long as I wanted. They have had to ask me to stop!

Over time their capacity usually increases though. Often it's just the skin getting used to so much friction. Otherwise they tell me when they can only tolerate ten or fifteen more minutes so I can get to a place where I actually **can** stop.

Sensitive skin isn't the only limiter for some women. Having that much pleasure with orgasms continuously building in intensity simply drives some women into an unbearable state. They simply have to stop. Or, they learn to surrender and move into a totally different state.

At this point, my path is very different. I'm more into the tantric aspect of sex. It is difficult to explain, and not appropriate for this book. Just know that there is huge diversity in sex that is so much more than just coupling to satisfy our animalistic urges with orgasms.

As mentioned, the following material is unique and very powerful. Study it often, and practice the techniques. There's always more to learn. One goal of mine is to present enough information here that you can continue to learn from your experiences as they deepen and expand.

Introduction to Locks

As already mentioned, locks literally lock the energy in the body. They do this in three different ways, one for each of the three locks.

Locks can be done in different ways. It is popular to teach the muscular method in yoga classes these days. That involves using muscular strength to make the lock happen.

Yoga exercises are even taught to strengthen that ability. Squeezing the PC muscle is one. However, a muscular lock only works to a point.

The most powerful way to do locks is to use a particular breathing technique. When that breathing technique is used the locks more or less happen by themselves. While muscles are involved, it's not the same at all. You are not doing the muscles, they work on their own which is **much** more powerful than the muscular method.

The Locks

The three locks are the genital/anal lock, the diaphragm lock and the throat lock. You have already learned the genital/anal lock muscular technique which is squeezing the PC muscle. When using the breathing technique the squeeze is much stronger than just willfully restraining an ejaculation like you have already learned.

As mentioned, the difference is that the root lock, as the PC squeeze is called in yoga, is done more or less spontaneously than strictly as an exercise. Ideally, when restraining, all the locks happen at the same time using the breathing technique as well as using some willful initiation.

The diaphragm lock, called the flying up lock in yoga, happens when the diaphragm area draws up and in. It can be extreme when using the breath work with the area drawing in more than you could do just by sucking that area in with your muscles. The throat lock is similar in that the hollow of the throat is drawn in strongly while the chin presses strongly down to the chest.

The purpose of the root lock is to drive the energy up, the diaphragm lock pulls the energy up and the throat lock keeps the energy from going back down. Ejaculatory restraint is almost completely insured when all three locks happen together at the right time.

Practicing the locks is done in various yoga postures. Generally, every yoga posture stimulates one or sometimes two of the seven energy centers called chakras.

However, some poses can stimulate more than one chakra. A few poses can even activate all seven chakras at once depending on the circumstances.

The breathing practice that causes the locks to occur spontaneously is holding an exhale. That is, you hold the breath out of the lungs. This can take a little practice since we are mostly used to holding our breath with the lungs full of air. It takes practice to get used to holding an exhale.

Holding an Exhale

Holding the air out of the lungs is counter to just about everything that is we normally do. And, it is important that **all** the air is pushed out of the lungs for the full experience.

Of course, it is not possible to hold the lungs empty nearly as long as holding them full, so it takes practice to get good at it. And, it takes practice to make sure that the last little bit of air is pushed out.

Also, because you won't be able to hold your exhale for more than a few seconds, there is a short window of time that ejaculation can be held back using this technique. Finding the right timing is essential. Practicing the yoga postures will give you the ability to hold your lungs empty longer which will increase the length of time you have to work with.

An important thing to understand is that the only postures that holding the exhale should be practiced with are the ones that stimulate the three lower chakras. You aren't likely to damage yourself if you do the wrong thing once or twice, but holding the exhale with different poses than recommended long term can cause problems.

The breathing specifics for each pose are very clear in the chapter on the yoga class.

Now that you know about locks, you can see if you can get one of more to apply when you practice muscular restraint. You'll need to initialize the lock willfully, but if you are holding an exhale you'll likely find it working within a few tries. The yoga class will increase your ability and insure the locks happen for you.

Start experimenting with the root lock when you practice the self-stimulation restraint. You can also experiment when having sex with your partner if you like.

Breath of Fire

Another yogic breathing technique that is used is the breath of fire. This is a rapid breathing technique that precedes the complete exhale, especially when holding back an ejaculation. Its purpose is to charge the body with oxygen so you can hold the exhale longer, as well as to charge the body with energy that helps strengthens your restraint.

While the breath of fire is done before exhaling completely to promote the locks and restraint, the initial practice is done includes holding the lungs full only. The full lung hold is also a good practice for generally giving you more energy.

The hold after doing breath of fire is done by squeezing your nostrils closed with your fingers, not by holding air in the lungs with your diaphragm and rib strength. This is pretty different too, but necessary because of the way the energy is charged into the body.

There are specific fingers to use with most yogic breathing techniques including the breath of fire. This is important for how the energy flows in the fingers to help with the flow of energy and to charge the body.

It probably wouldn't matter if you didn't do the right fingering technique a couple dozen times, but you really need to do a lot more than that for best results. So, try your best to get used to the fingering early.

To start the breath of fire, take a deep full breath in through your nose. Make sure you suck in every last bit of air that you can, and hold your breath for just a few seconds. Hold for no more than ten seconds, otherwise you can get out of breath. Then exhale fully releasing the air out through your mouth.

Let your next inhale be natural filling your lungs to a neutral level, where they would fill to when relaxed and not breathing. Then, use rapid diaphragm contractions to create short sharp exhales. Let the inhale happen when you relax the diaphragm after the air is pushed out from the contraction that made you exhale. Immediately compress your diaphragm again, let the air relax in again, and continue.

Do about 30 of these contractions before closing off your right nostril with your right thumb and inhale deeply through the left nostril. Take that inhale right after your last compression exhale.

Hold your breath by pinching your nose tightly with your right thumb on your right nostril, and the right hand middle and ring finger on your left nostril.

Remember, you're holding your breath by holding your nose. If you were to release your fingers air would rush out. The lungs, diaphragm and ribs need to be completely relaxed with this hold.

Hold your breath as long as you comfortably can and exhale with control through your mouth after releasing your fingers. You don't want to push holding your breath so that you are gasping for breath and have to hurry the exhale when you release, though you should be just a little out of breath when done.

Take however many normalizing breaths you need until you are breathing normally again, then do the breath of fire again.

Another way to get the idea of how to do the contractions for the exhale is to suddenly push your upper belly just below the diaphragm so the breath is pushed out. Or, have a friend push the area for you. It shouldn't hurt, just enough push to push the air out of your relaxed lungs.

Most people start doing breath of fire with slow contractions which is fine. The contractions and inhale will get faster with practice. I can do 30 contractions in less than five seconds; a beginner might take 15 or 20 seconds.

If you are confused, you might try finding a video how it is done. Check kalidasa.com to see if I have a video on how to do this. Or, check YouTube if I haven't gotten one up yet.

Start with five repetitions and build up to around 30. More is ok if you really get into it. 30 is great, but most people won't stick with it long term because it can be really intense. The main place you will be using the breath of fire is while restraining your ejaculation.

Another benefit of the breath of fire is that it helps to rid the body of toxins. But, there is a caution you need to know about.

The detoxification, as well as the extra oxygenation that comes with the breath of fire, can leave you feeling a bit spacey. So, avoid driving or doing anything potentially dangerous after breath of fire until you know how you are affected by it. Wait at least 30 minutes to an hour.

Regular practice of breath of fire is a great way to charge your body as well as to help eliminate toxins which can sap energy. Best of all, that extra internal energy will help you restrain ejaculations in general.

Practicing breath of fire just before restraint will give you even more strength for that herculean task. There are more details on that to come.

Inducing Your First Lock

The yoga practice below is a great way to encourage the locks and get you started on using that technique for restraining ejaculations. But, your first experience of a lock may be difficult. Here is a simple posture that works well for giving people their first experience of a lock.

The lock we're going to try for is the second one, the flying up lock (diaphragm lock). You'll be doing the lock in a muscular why while holding an exhale.

The energy that will drive the lock should take over before you need to inhale. It will likely get stronger as you get closer to needing to inhale. Inhale sooner if you need to, you can always practice it again. It will usually happen within a few tries.

The pose is standing with your feet hip width or more apart, your knees slightly bent with your hands on your knees. Try to keep your weight in your feet, but you can lean on your knees if you need to. Relax as much as you can throughout.

Take a deep breath and exhale all the air out. Be sure to push out all the air you can. Push one last time to get that last bit!

Then, while holding your exhale, pull your diaphragm area in. Sucking your belly in is another way to think about it. Hold until you need to inhale again.

You don't need to push it. You can practice as much as you like to find out how long it works for you to hold an exhale.

You should notice the body automatically trying to pull your stomach in, especially your upper stomach. It may only happen right before you need to inhale.

After a few tries it should pull in on its own before you at least a couple of seconds before you need to inhale. With more practice you will be able to push the length of time you can hold the exhale simply because you will know what it feels like -- it can be a bit weird at first!

You may notice something else too. It's good to notice what happens internally as well as externally when doing any yoga technique. Usually, an inner peace comes over people for a few moments before they need to inhale. It can be the most impressive part of the practice.

Practice a few times, especially if the lock isn't happening for you. It is a good idea to practice a few times even if you get the lock right away so that you prepare yourself for doing the locks in the yoga class.

Introduction to the Yoga Class

This short yoga class is designed to bring the energy up the body. It is called Energy Yoga because it energizes the body in an amazing way.

One of the high priority teachings in yoga is about ethics. That is because people develop certain abilities while on the path to Truth. And, unethical behavior causes a loss in that endeavor.

How that happens is individual. The point is, if you abuse any power you will feel guilty on a higher level, and you will actually hold yourself back.

This book, especially this yoga class, teaches how to gain powerful abilities that can give you power over others. It is very tempting to go out and have a great time at the expense of others. However, if you do, there will be an opposite reaction.

What ethics should you follow? Yoga offers specific advice, but it really comes down to what you already know in your heart to be right or wrong.

One way to gauge is to notice if you are treating people better today than you did in the recent past. Perhaps you learn a lesson, someone gets hurt, and so you change how you do things. You have progressed! And, your abilities will progress as well.

I offer this piece of advice because I feel a certain responsibility to you, my reader, because I am teaching very powerful piece of what I have learned through decades of growth through yoga. And, because I have learned some very hard lessons that following this simple advice would have made much easier.

Now, let's get back to the some yoga that will help increase all your abilities.

There are several poses that can be used for each of the seven energy centers, but only two each are presented here. Just about everyone will be able to do at least one of the poses.

There are a lot of ways to modify a pose if there is some sort of physical limitation. See if you can find a slight modification that works for you if you need to. You can also ask a yoga instructor to help with your particular limitation.

According to yoga physiology there are seven energy centers called chakras. Each has its own energy, color, god and more. In this case we are interested in their energy, and how to move that energy up the chain of chakras using yoga postures and breathing techniques.

There are countless yoga postures. Each one will stimulate one or two chakras, sometimes more. This stimulation is greatly increased when a posture is combined with the appropriate breathing practices.

It is important to focus your attention on the energy center associated with the pose you are doing. Your attention will help move the energy up your body. Keep your attention focused on the area as you do the recommended breathing practice.

The breathing practices used are either to hold a deep breath with the lungs full, hold an exhale with the lungs empty or diaphragmatic breathing.

A lot of times the breath may shift from diaphragmatic breathing to just breathing normally. This is actually quite normal because breathing practices will bring up and clear early life trauma which we tend to avoid because of the pain.

When you notice your breath change, simply notice what is going on internally and go back to the technique. You may find yourself moving through issues that hold you back in life. That is a big part of why breathing practices are so powerful.

If holding the breath in is called for in the pose you would take a deep three part breath to hold, usually after breathing diaphragmatically in the pose for three to five breaths.

The three part breath is filling the lungs from the belly up. It starts with a diaphragmatic breath, with the breath then filling the solar plexus area and then your chest last.

If the pose calls for holding an exhale you would take three to five normal breaths in the pose before blowing all your air out and holding the breath out of your lungs, an empty lung hold. Be sure to do a final squeeze to remove the last bit of air so that your lungs are completely empty.

The root chakra is the most important of them all. That is true of this class and in general as well. It is the root of the energy needed to restrain an ejaculation.

The root lock is associated with the root chakra. It is similar to the PC muscle exercise in that the genital/anal area is drawn up. However, the strength of a lock done with the right breath is much greater than when the area is drawn up as an exercise.

There are poses for all the energy centers in the class below, two poses for each chakra. You only need to do one for each chakra.

For a longer yoga practice and for greater benefit you can do them all. An option if you can't do one of the poses is to repeat the one you can do. You can also hold the pose longer by repeating the breathing technique more than recommended for even more benefit.

Remember though, this class can make you spacy. So, be careful not to do anything dangerous after.

The first time I did a practice like this I got so wigged out that I didn't know how out of it I was. My fellow student and I were laughing at the most ridiculous things. We were complete fools! What fun we had!

I don't even remember driving after that, but I'm sure I must have. Not the best idea looking back.

It is possible for all the locks to occur with the first three sets of poses. That is, for the first three chakras which are the lower three chakras. However, only one or even none may happen for you the first few times you do the class.

The instructions for the poses say that you can induce the locks. That is, you can squeeze the PC muscle, draw your belly strongly in and to tuck your chin as you draw your throat in.

The locks will usually happen when you get close to the maximum time you can hold your breath out. Eventually the locks will happen by themselves. They will also start happening sooner after holding your exhale. So, try the technique without inducing from time to time to see if you're there yet.

There is an energy focus included with each pose. The pairs of poses each have different foci. While the energies may seem different, they still both relate to the chakra being stimulated by the pose. You can choose the one that strikes closer to home for you, or change as you like.

If you are single, you can focus on the partner you desire, or on the one you are seeking where it says to focus on your partner.

Yoga means union with the Divine. These poses combined with the breathing technique will burn off the impurities that keep that union from happening. That includes the union with a loving partner with a Divine component.

The process of clearing the way from you having union with a partner is a burning up, or clearing, of the barriers that keep you from her. This burning is called the yogic fire where impurities are destroyed.

Each chakra has negative as well as a positive emotions associated with it. The negative emotions may come up as you stimulate the chakras with the pose and breathe.

This is an example of yogic burning where impurities are burned up in the fires of yoga (union). Rejoice if this happens to you! It means you are getting closer to your partner!

Allow this burning to happen during any of the practices in this book. It may be uncomfortable in the moment, but the improvement in your relationships that comes after is well worth it.

Energy Yoga Class

Half Lotus -- Root Chakra

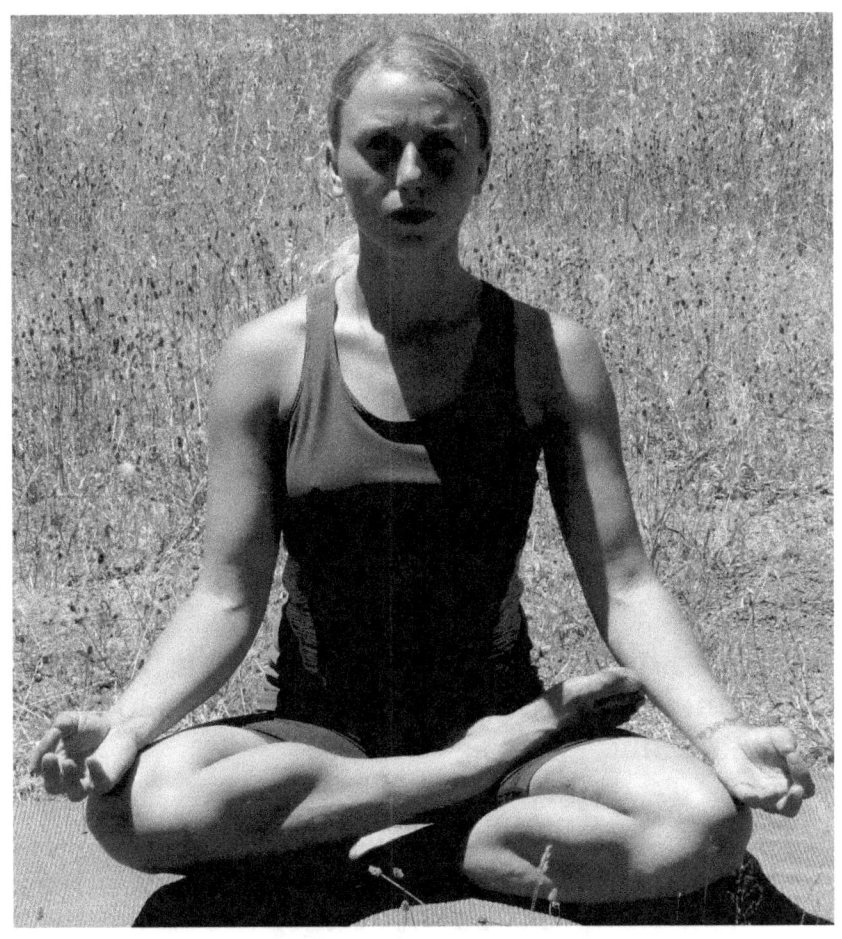

The root chakra is located in the perineum. It's also associated with the bottom of spine. It holds the energy of survival. Animals are that they will survive. We human animals will always strive to find a way to survive no matter what place or condition we may find ourselves in. This drive comes from the root chakra.

It also holds Divine energy in that it is one end of our connection to the Divine. The connection between it and the crown chakra is our connection to the Divine. Stimulating the energy of the root chakra stimulates the connection to what you consider to be perfect.

One of the best yoga postures to activate the root chakra is the half lotus. When done correctly the energy of this center is kicked off in a very strong way.

Lotus and half lotus are unique poses in that they can stimulate all the chakras. They can also stimulate all the locks.

For a lot of people lotus is hard to do, but half lotus can be done by most people. It doesn't matter which foot is on top, either position will stimulate the first chakra.

Half lotus is done sitting on one foot so that the heel is pressed into the perineum. Place the sole of the foot along the opposite thigh, not under.

The outside of the foot can be slightly under the thigh though. Most beginners tend to tuck the foot in further sitting on it, avoid that.

The opposite leg is placed on top so you are in a crossed legged position. The backs of the wrists are placed on the knees with the palms up. Lightly connect the thumb and forefinger. Relax your shoulder and arms for maximum energy flow.

Keep your spine tall in the pose with your chin down slightly so the back of the neck is slightly flattened. Ideally you would not be leaning against anything because that can interfere with the flow of energy up the spine. However, it is more important to have a straight and tall spine, so lightly lean against something if you really need to.

A modified version can be done with the opposite leg extended straight out if there is anything preventing you from crossing your legs. If that is the case, take a minute whenever you practice half lotus to stretch that leg on top until you can sit comfortably in the pose.

Take two or three diaphragmatic breaths in the pose. Then, take a full breath followed by exhaling all the air out of your lungs. Push to get the last bit out, and hold the air out of your lungs as long as you comfortably can.

Focus your attention on the root chakra, where your heel is pressing. Focus on the energy that keeps you going as you hold the exhale.

Notice if depression, or a loss of interest in life, like you'd rather not actively participate in life, comes to your consciousness while holding this pose. Allow the emotion to be burned up as your mind reaches the peaceful place that comes when holding an exhale.

At first, you can induce all the locks as you hold your breath out. From time to time practice without inducing them to see if they happen on their own.

Take as many recovery breaths as you need to normalize your breathing. Switch your legs around so the top leg is below and the lower leg is above and repeat the breathing technique and locks.

You can do several repetitions if you like, but it is best to start with one on each side until you find out how this technique affects you. Keep a balance with which leg is on top as the pressure of the foot on the thigh influences the energy channels which need to be kept balanced.

Lotus -- Root Chakra

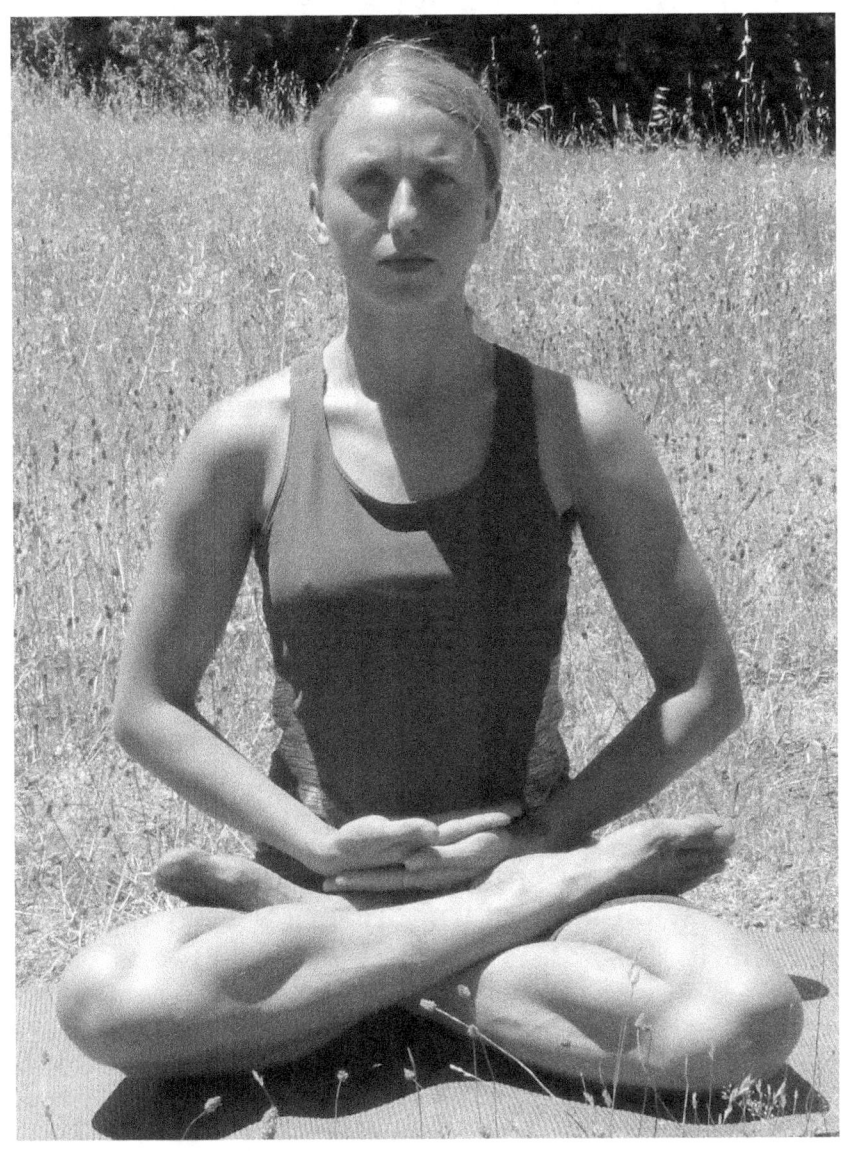

Lotus is a pose that will simple be impossible for some. The reason I include it here is because there are great benefits for those that can.

The pose is done by placing one leg over the other so the feet are pressing on the thighs. The hands are placed one over the other with the same hand on top as the leg that is on top, palms turned up and stacked over each other.

Take a few diaphragmatic breaths, then inhale fully and exhale completely holding the exhale as you focus on your perineum. You can induce all the locks as you hold your breath out.

The other root energy you can focus on has to do with your connection to the Divine. Notice how it drives up your spine to awaken your inner light.

One of the extra benefits comes from your feet pressing on your thighs. This causes both energy and blood to be pushed up to the genitals. That increase in flow helps keep the energy moving up which is what is most important for restraining ejaculation.

Lotus is one of the best poses for activating all three locks. The energy really likes to move upward in lotus. Practicing either lotus or half lotus alone is a good way to get at least some great energy activation happening if you are limited on time.

Bound Angle --Sex Center

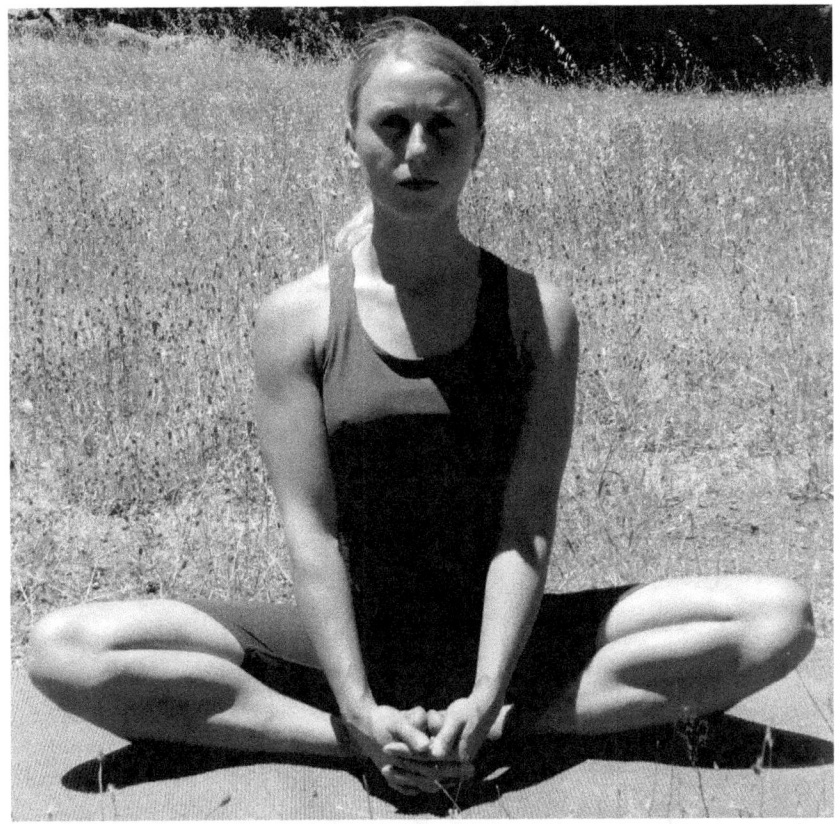

The second chakra is located from just above the perineum, or base of the genitals, to the top of the genitals, or just below the pubic bone.

The second chakra includes the genitals which have to do with reproduction. Giving and receiving intense pleasure is what insures the race will continue. We are driven by pleasure to have sex and reproduce. This urge is the most powerful force in the universe.

Activating the sexual center in this class is just a step in bringing the energy up. It is important to do the rest of the class once you activate this center, or the energy could come crashing down.

Bound angle is done by placing the soles of the feet together. Interlace your fingers and wrap your hands wrapped around the feet. Use the arm strength to draw the lower back in and make the spine tall. Drop your chin slightly so the back of the neck is as flat as possible.

Keep the elbows and shoulders down with the shoulders relaxed in such a way that the only active part of the arms is the bicep muscles. Activate your legs to work the knees toward the floor. Relax every part of your body that is not involved in the stretch.

Keeping the spine tall in the above position is difficult for some people. If that is the case, you can put your hands behind your back palms on the floor with the fingers pointing back. Press the hands to make your spine tall.

Most people will do this best with the arms pressed tight against the back. Having the fingers pointed forward is okay if that is more comfortable for you.

A flat back is important, having the hands further back to accommodate that is fine even if you lean back slightly at the waist, as long as your back is straight.

Take a few diaphragmatic breaths in the pose, and then inhale fully to exhale completely and hold the exhale. You can induce all the locks as you hold your breath out.

Focus on your genital area and the intensity you experience with your partner during the reproductive act.

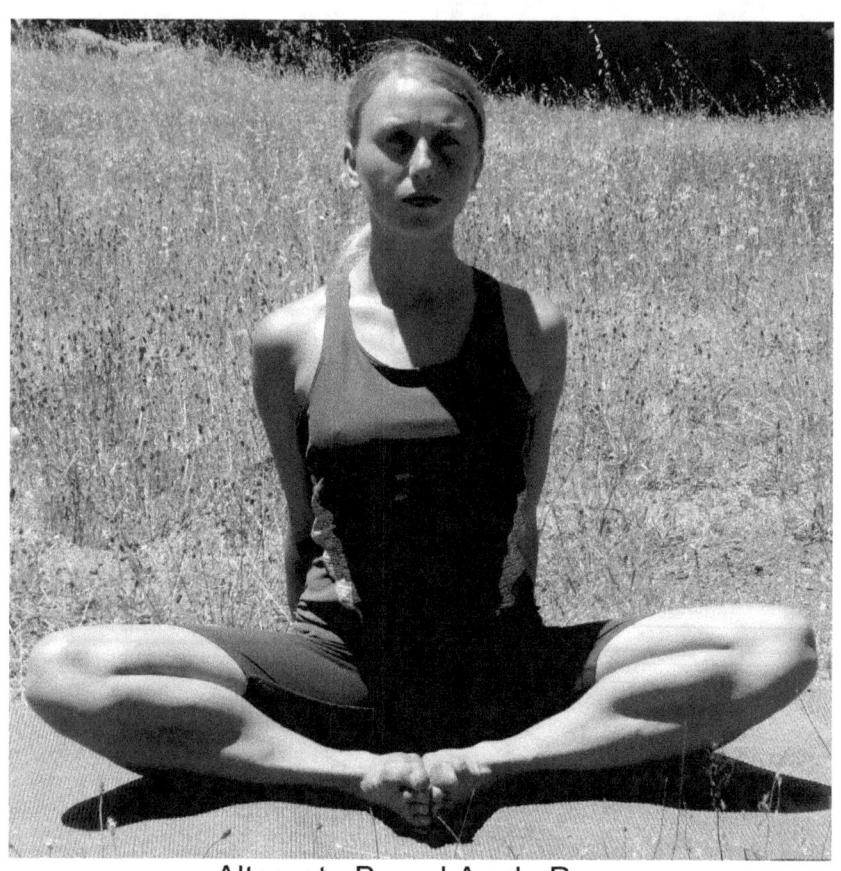

Alternate Bound Angle Pose

Angle Asana -- Sex Center

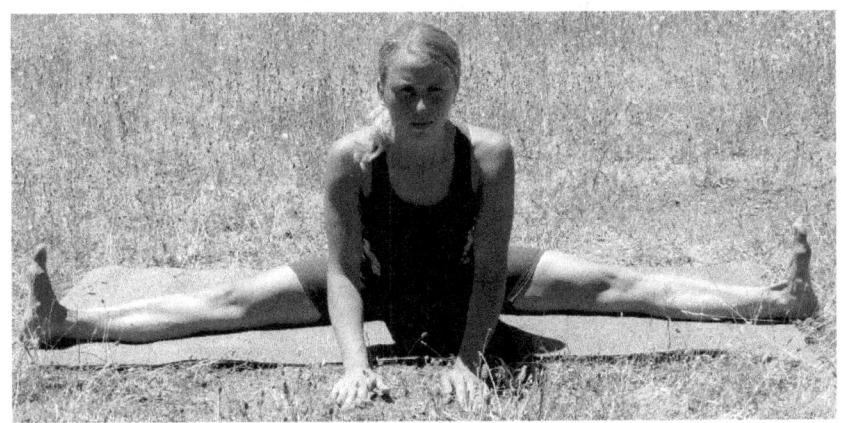

This is a great stretch for the groin (gracilis) and backs of the thighs. This can really help you be a better lover because of it increases blood flow to the genital area for a stronger erection.

The pose is done by sitting with your legs spread wide and leaning forward. Rotate your thighs back by trying to point your toes back behind you, at least in that direction. Reach forward as far as you can and breathe in the area that is stretching.

Allow the area to soften and warm up with gentle diaphragmatic breathing. Your body will naturally rise as you inhale and release as you exhale. Allow this movement to help with the stretch.

After a few breaths in the pose, take a deep breath and exhale all the air from your lungs. Focus on your genital area as you hold the breath and allow or induce the first lock. Notice the energy of reproduction, especially if you are trying for a child. Or, notice how the energy to reproduce drives you to seek the pleasure of a loving partner.

With practice the other locks may occur as well. You can induce them from time to time to see if they might activate on their own.

Some people will be much more flexible in this pose than others. There are things that can be done for different ability levels. For less flexible people, holding a strap around each foot is very helpful. If you can, reach out and hold your feet to pull yourself into the stretch.

If you can go deep into the pose you may prefer to reach your hands out in front of you. Let the reach pull you into the stretch, and let your breath help your body forward and down. Very limber people will need to very actively roll their thighs back for the best stretch.

Sitting Twist -- Power Center

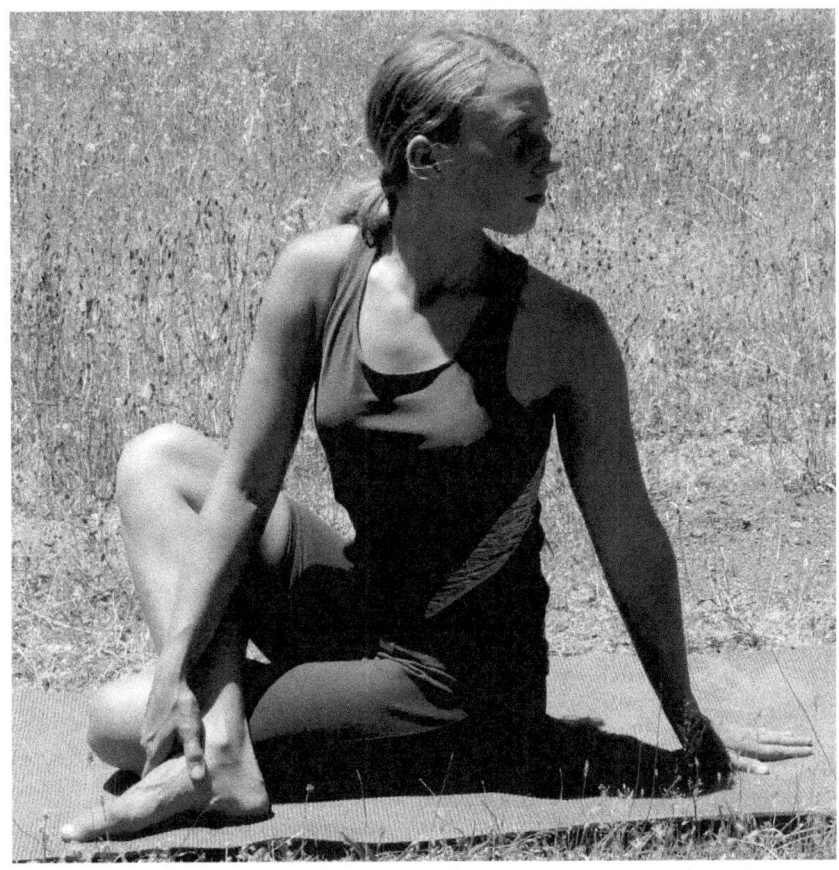

The third chakra is centered just below the belly button and extends up to the diaphragm. It has to do with power. It takes great personal power to pull the sexual energy up to this area.

This also creates more personal power. This power can be used to satisfy life's many desires.

Lovers, fighters, business people, parents and more all direct this power in their own way.

Start by sitting with both legs extended. Take your right foot over your left leg and place the sole on the ground. One option is to keep the left leg extended. The other is to take the left foot up to your right hip, not under. The right sit bone needs to go to the floor. If it doesn't go all the way down, or if you tend to tip over unless you hold yourself up, you are better off keeping the right leg straight. You'll get the same benefit.

Take your right arm over the left leg and place it between the leg and your body. Hold your left foot with it. Place your left hand on the floor near your right foot.

With an inhale, take your left arm up bringing your hand to eye level. As you exhale rotate your body taking your hand back behind you and place it on the floor behind your left hip. Use your hand on the floor and the arm pressing against your leg to help draw you deeply into the twist.

Take a few diaphragmatic breaths in the pose. As you inhale you will naturally rotate slightly out of the pose, as you exhale you will naturally be able to rotate more deeply into the twist. You can pull into the twist with the exhales for the best twist. After three or so breaths exhale completely as you draw yourself strongly into the stretch and hold the exhale.

As you hold the exhale, focus your attention on your lower belly. Notice the power you have to fulfill your life's desires.

Come out of the pose by bring your back arm up and rotating forward out of the pose as you inhale. Repeat the pose and breathing technique on the other side. You can repeat the pose on both sides for maximum benefit.

This and the next twist will specifically stimulate the diaphragm lock. But, all the poses in which you hold the exhale can simulate all three locks simultaneously.

Reclining Twist -- Power Center

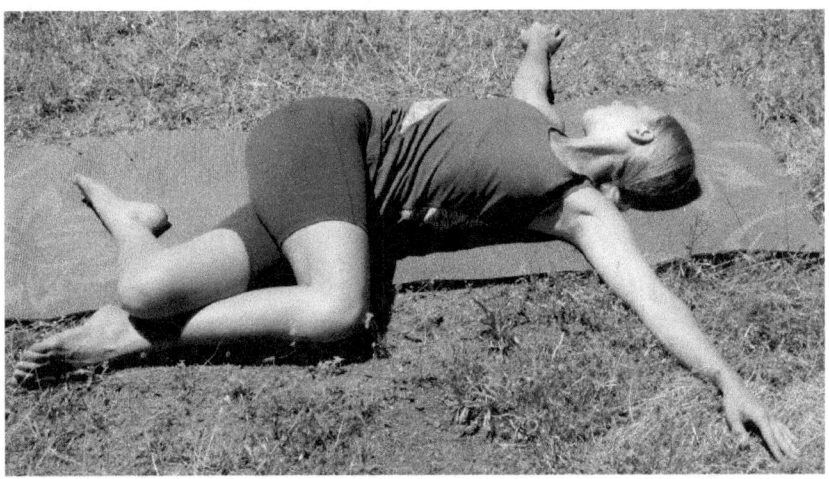

Start by lying on your back with your knees bent, feet on the floor. Cross your right leg over the left so your legs are crossed. Drop your legs to the left coming into the twist. Shift your hips around so you are fully into the twist with your right knee on the floor. Spread your arms to the side and turn your head to the right so you are looking toward your right hand.

Your right shoulder blade should be off the floor. If not, bring your right hand to the left to roll onto your left side, and shift your hips further around so the shoulder blade is lifted when you take your right hand back to the right to spread your arms back open.

As you breathe in the pose your right shoulder blade will rise and fall with your breath. After a few diaphragmatic breaths inhale fully, then exhale completely and relax in the twist as you hold your exhale.

Focus your attention on the third chakra in your lower belly. Be with the energy of joy and generosity as you go into the peace that comes with holding an exhale.

The emotion that is purified in the third chakra is jealousy. Notice it if it comes up and allow it to release.

Inhale as you come out of the pose. Complete the sequence by doing the pose on the other side. Repeat the two sides for full benefit.

Serpent -- Heart Center

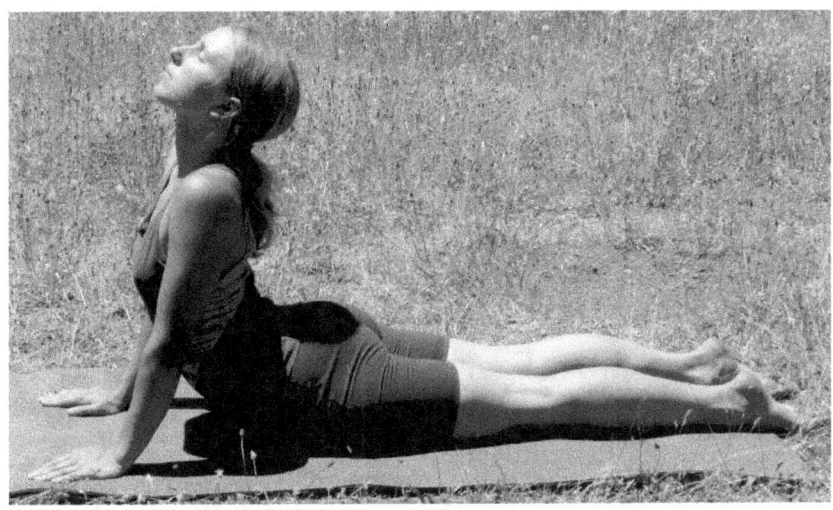

The fourth energy center is the heart chakra which is centered in the solar plexus just below the breastbone. It extends up to just below the hollow of the throat. The entire chest area is considered the heart chakra as are the arms, especially when used in a loving embrace.

This energy center has to do with divine love, which is defined as loving for no reason at all. The warm feeling of love you feel in your chest when you think of someone dear, like your lover, is divine in nature.

There are several variations of serpent pose. Straight arm serpent is the best pose for activating the heart. An alternate that is still a powerful heart chakra activator is sometimes called the sphinx pose is done with the elbows and forearms on the floor with the elbows right under your shoulders.

Start lying flat on your belly, palms under your shoulders with your legs together. Separating the legs slightly is fine. Take a deep breath, as you exhale press your hands into the floor lifting your upper body by straightening your arms.

There is a tendency to let the body slouch down so the head drops towards the shoulders. Keep activating the pose by lifting your body up out of the shoulders during the pose. Remember, this is a strong pose to bring strength and energy into your body.

Take a few diaphragmatic breaths in the pose. Have your final inhale be a full breath and hold your breath as you put your attention on your heart chakra. Focus the loving feelings you have toward your loving partner while holding the breath and pose.

The emotion that pulls the heart energy down is jealousy. Notice if it comes to consciousness and realize that it can destroy relationships. Allow it to burn as you remember the love you share with your partner.

Release down out of the pose as you release your breath. Repeat the pose and breathing.

If you do the pose on your forearms you can hold the pose rather than releasing with the exhale. Hold an inhale two or three times while you hold the pose. Take a couple of normalizing breaths in between.

Camel -- Heart Center

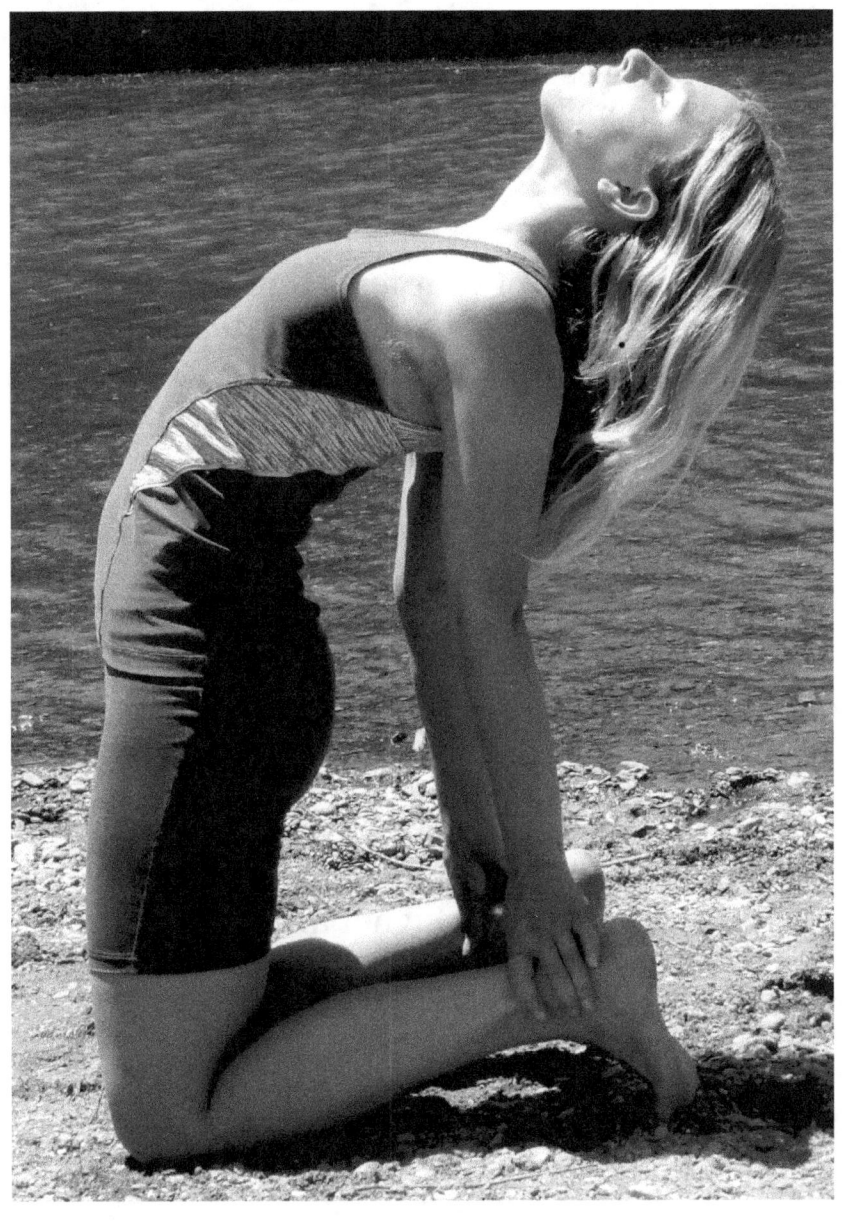

There are several variations of camel pose that can make it easier for people with less backbend ability. You can use blocks, or whatever you have available, to put your hands on so your body is taller and in less of an arch is one of the best ways to help make camel pose easier without sacrificing benefit.

The best way to do that with blocks is to place one on either side of your feet to give you something to put your hands on instead of reaching all the way to your feet. The blocks are usually nine inches tall, but a taller prop is fine to use if you need more help. Placing your elbows on a chair behind you is another possibility.

Start in an upright kneeling position. Use padding under your knees as needed. Take a deep breath and exhale as you reach back taking your hands to your heels. Press your thighs away from you to activate the pose and open your chest and heart chakra.

The easiest way to do camel pose is to be up on your toes so your heels higher and easier to reach. If you have a good back bend you can have your feet flat so the tops are on the floor.

There may be a temptation to reach one hand back to one foot at a time. It is much better to reach straight back into the pose because the twist and arch can be hard on your back and could even cause injury.

After a few diaphragmatic breaths in the pose take a deep inhale and hold your breath. Bring loving energy and attention to your heart chakra. Contemplate on the joy and generosity that bubbles forth from the heart chakra.

Release the pose by inhaling as you come up, or simply sit down, especially if that is easier on your back.

Another variation that is easy on the back is to exhale back with your hands on your hips/lower back area rather than reaching all the way down to your feet. Once in the pose lift your chest high to open your heart chakra as you hold your inhale.

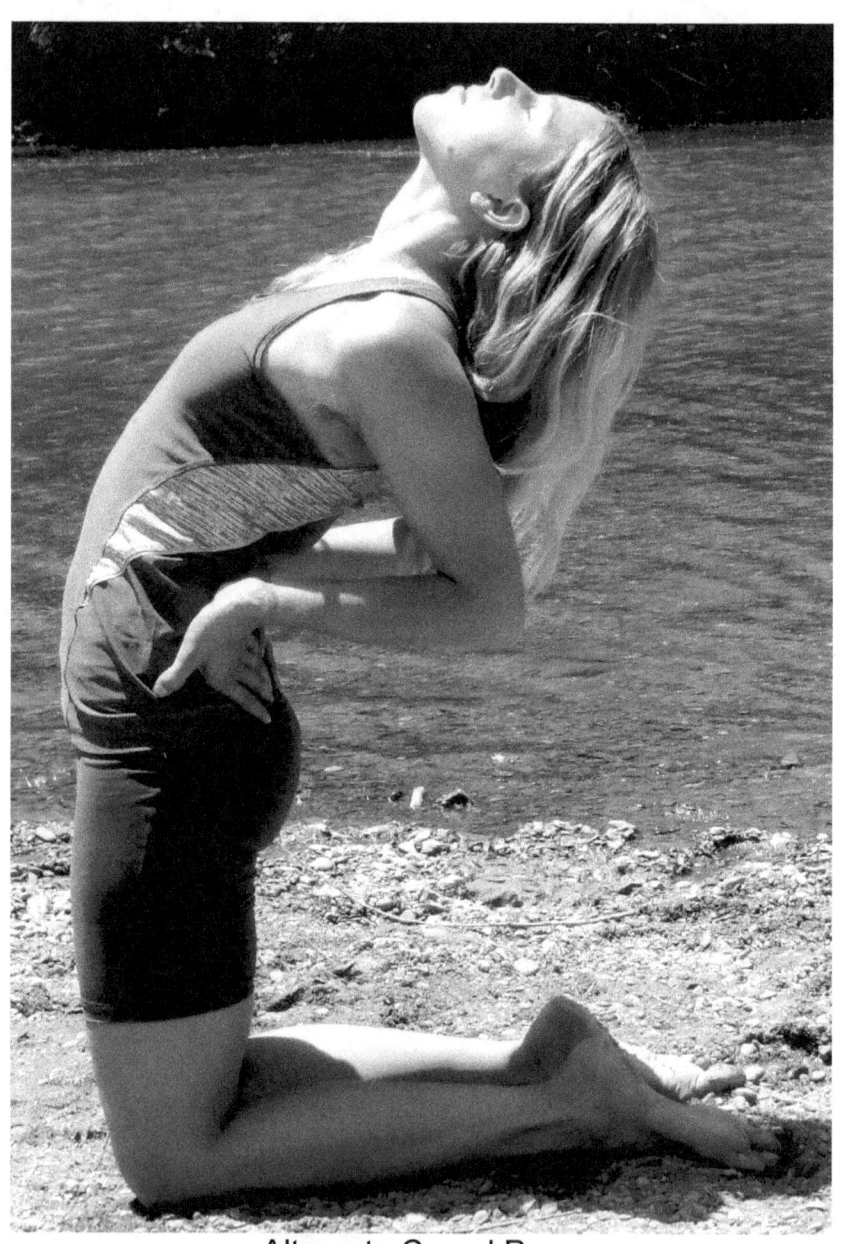

Alternate Camel Pose

Plough/Half Plough -- Throat Center

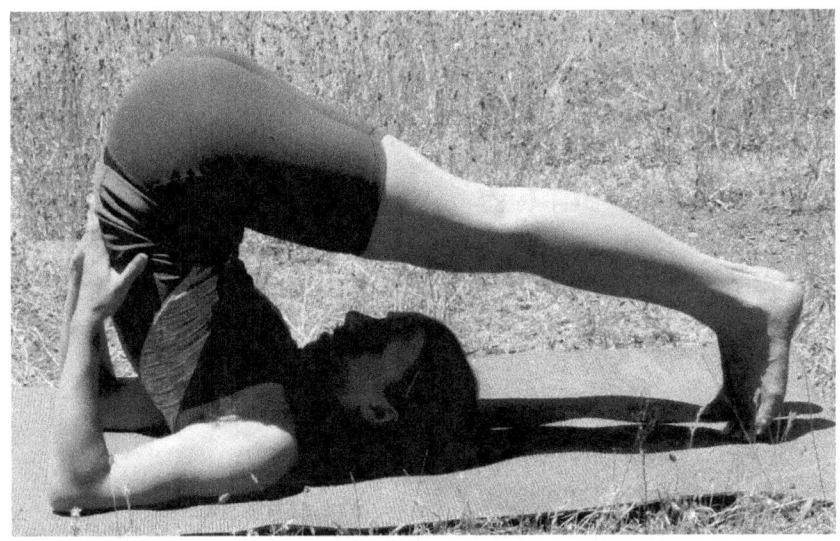

The fifth chakra is the throat chakra. It has to do with speaking your truth, saying how things truly are for you, especially messages of love. And, it has to do with keeping integrity with whoever you are in relationship with, especially your lover.

By speaking up for yourself it can be a form of taking back your power from others who may have done or said things to take power from you. However, that can also be done in an angry way, which brings the throat energy down.

The chakra's root is in the hollow of the throat. It extends to between the eyebrows and includes the throat, neck and all of the face up to the forehead.

Plough pose can be a little hard on the neck because of the compression it puts on the vertebral discs. You can either skip this pose if you have a neck problem, or use folded blankets under your shoulders to take pressure off your neck. Half plough is another option for neck issues since the compression is much less than what happens in plough.

Start lying on your back. Lift your hips and legs so your legs come overhead and down behind you so your toes are resting overhead on the floor. Place your hands on your back for support. Reach your hips toward the ceiling to make the lower back as flat as you can.

For half plough, bring your legs overhead without taking your feet to the floor. Support yourself with your hands on your back. Keep your hips low so the back is rounded. That way your neck has little to no pressure on it.

You can also try the advanced half plough by placing your hands on your thighs just above the knees. Ideally, you would keep your arms straight as you balance on your shoulders.

The balance can be difficult. Shifting your shoulders around for a better base can be very helpful. Also, you can have a friend hold your legs while you adjust your shoulders and find your balance.

Another variation is to put a chair behind you to rest your feet on.

Some people find these poses very comfortable, but have trouble kicking their legs up overhead. Try coming into the pose with your hips near a wall and your head pointing away from the wall. Walk your feet up the wall to get your hips up and gently bring one leg overhead at a time to come into the pose. For even more help, place a chair at the wall so you can put your feet on the seat to help you up into the pose.

The breathing for half plough is diaphragmatic breathing without a hold. The breath can also be deeper, moving toward the three part breath as your ability increases.

The attention is usually on the hollow of the throat, but can go to anywhere in the throat chakra area your attention happens to go. Focus on your throat area as you breathe in the pose.

Think on keeping the flow of truth with your partner and others in your life. Or, meditate on the truth you endeavor to always share with your lover.

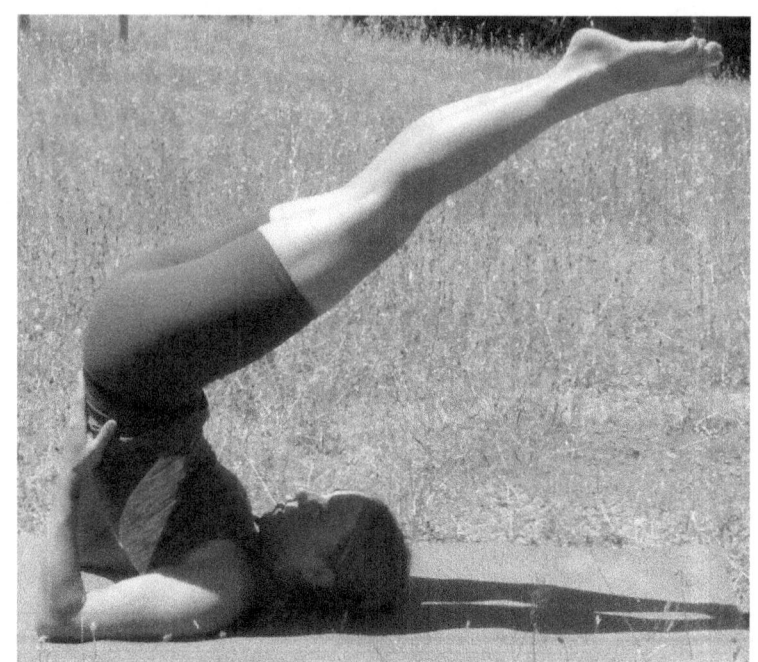

Half Plough Pose

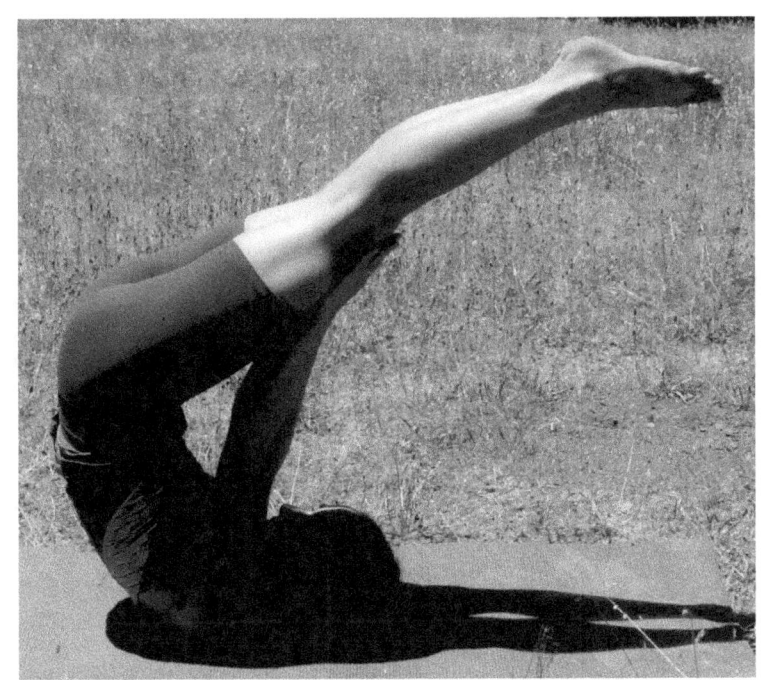

More Difficult Half Plough Pose

Half Fish -- Throat Chakra

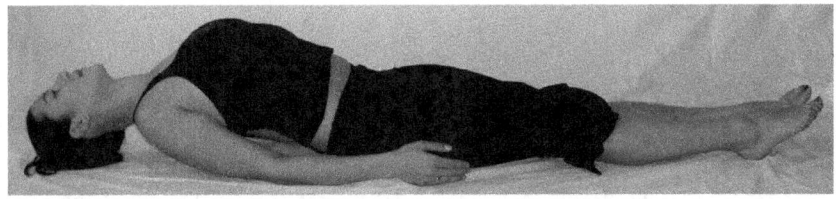

Half fish and plough pose are complimentary poses in that they offer a counter stretch for the main area that is worked. In plough pose, the neck is opened in back, but with some compression from the body's weight.

Half fish provides the opposite stretch on the neck with little or no weight so the neck is released from the compression caused by plough. Ideally you would always follow plough pose with a counter pose like half fish.

Start lying on your back, legs extended and together, arms by your side. With an exhale press your chest up using your arm strength to lift you onto your elbows.

Let your head roll back so the crown moves toward the floor. Avoid overarching your neck so you don't compress the vertebrae in back. A little less than a full arch of your neck is ideal.

Keep your weight in your arms rather than resting very much weight on your head. Only allow the weight of your head to rest on your head to keep from injuring yourself.

There is an advanced technique where the head holds the upper body off the floor, but that isn't necessary to activate the throat chakra. Only do the advanced technique if you are sure of your neck health. In that case, your hands would come into prayer position at the middle of your chest, and your legs would lift.

Take a few diaphragmatic breaths in the pose as you focus your attention on the throat chakra, wherever it is that you experience the energy. If you don't have a clear experience then keep your attention in the hollow of your throat as you increase the depth of your breath.

Increase the depth of your breath as you advance in this practice or as the energy moves you. It can increase from a diaphragmatic breath up to a full three part breath.

Repeat the pose and breathing technique two or three times. Focus on allowing the flow of Truth in your life as you hold the pose. Notice if any anger shows up to pull your energy down.

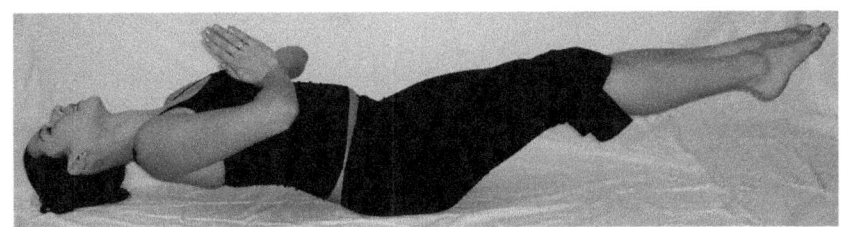

Advanced Half Fish

Childs Pose -- Third Eye

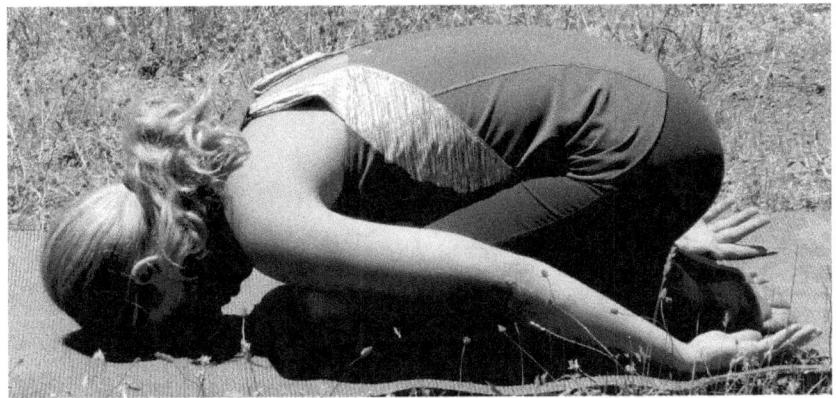

The root of the sixth chakra, the third eye, is located between the eyebrows. It extends up to the crown of the head which includes the entire brain area except for the lowest part of the pituitary gland and the very top of the brain. It is associated with inner sight, and awareness of the Divine which is seeing through the illusion of life.

Childs pose is a very relaxing pose that gives you the opportunity to focus on the third eye and its properties. However, knee problems can cause pain that can break your attention.

That can be helped by putting a blanket between your butt and heels rather than sitting directly on the heels. Use as much elevation as you need to avoid pain.

Start by sitting on your heels (or blanket), and bend forward to rest your forehead on the floor in front of you. Use padding for your head if you like.

Your arms either can either be extended out in front of you, or placed alongside your body. Try both, but realize that one may be best for you one day while the other may be more comfortable another time.

The breathing is a normal diaphragmatic breath throughout the time you hold the pose. Keep your attention on your third eye while relaxing and breathing in the pose.

Relax and focus on the Divine light that is your lover for one to three minutes, longer if you really enjoy the experience. You can deepen your breath if you are feeling more energized, or use a more relaxed breath if you are feeling more relaxed and focused.

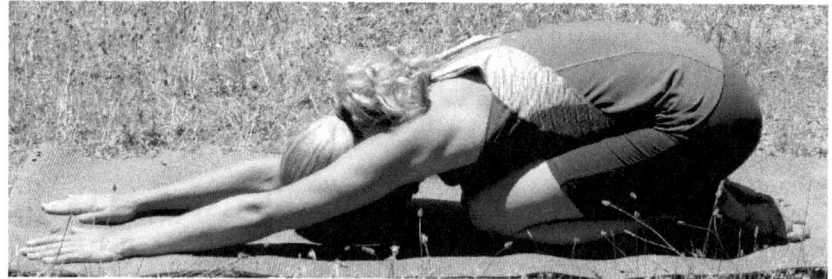

Childs Pose Arms Extended

Yoga Mudra -- Third Eye

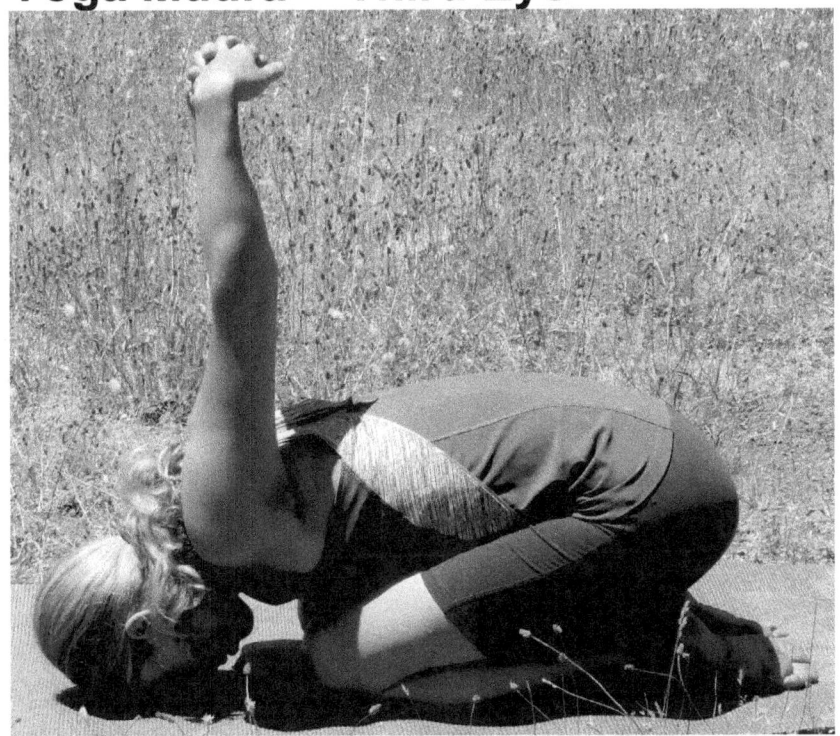

Yoga mudra is very similar to child's pose, but with a different arm position and activation. The name means "union seal." This is a mudra (seal) that comes from union (yoga) that seals the energy in the body.

Because it is a mudra it is more powerful than child's pose, and can be more energizing. Both are good for the third eye though, so chose the one that is best for you, or practice both in the order presented for more benefit.

Start in child's pose. Take your hands behind your back, interlace the fingers and draw your arms up overhead as far as you comfortably can. Palms down is generally the prescribed position, but turning the hands over is fine if that works for you.

Practice diaphragmatic breathing in the pose. You can allow the breaths to become fairly deep as your energy flows. Allow your arms to move as your breath moves your body.

Your breathing may charge your body with energy causing you to increase the stretch in the arms by bringing them further overhead. Or, you may feel like reaching your arms more strongly up and away from you. This is a good place to find yourself in, it means that your energy is awakening in your body and driving the poses.

Keep your attention on your third eye. Generally this will be between your eyebrows, but it can be in any area of the third eye, even a more internal area of your brain or head.

Keep your focus on what is really real in the world which is your relationship with the Divine. Remember that is your partner as well.

Frustration and even anger at not always having awareness of the Divine can bring the energy of the third eye down. Or, there may be anger toward your lover that is due to not being aware of the goddess that she is. Become aware of it and relax as you release from the burden.

Half Head Stand -- Crown Chakra

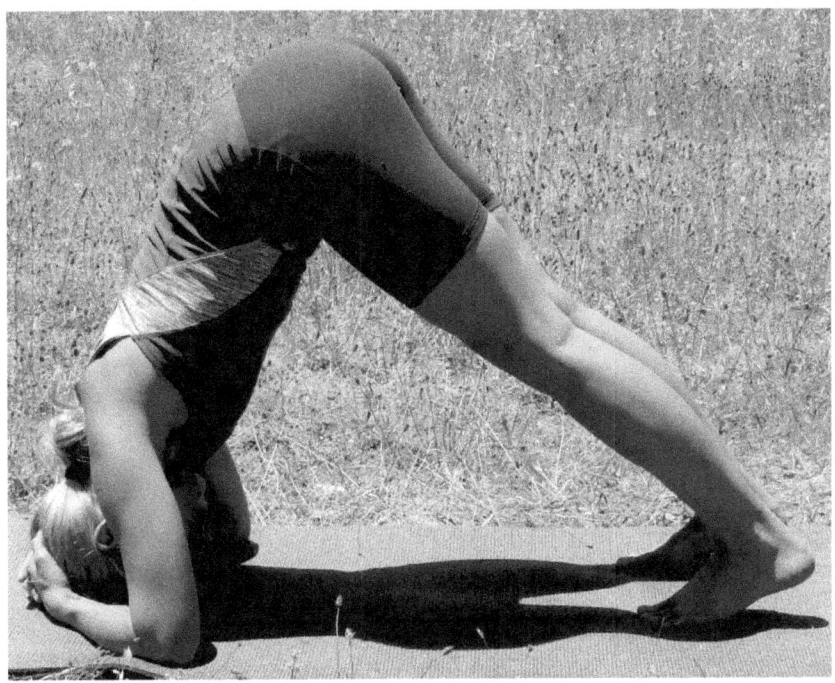

The crown chakra, the seventh and last chakra, is an area three to four inches in diameter centering on the very crown of your head. It has to do with enlightenment, or seeing the Truth of what really is.

There is a deep Divine experience when this chakra is fully awakened. In the practice here there can be an experience of high energy once the energy has been lifted to the crown.

The crown chakra is sometimes associated with either the pituitary or pineal gland depending on which system you reference. Physically it is centered at the top of the head above the pituitary gland which is more or less in the bottom center of the brain.

Energizing the crown chakra with yoga poses can be difficult as headstand is the ideal pose. However, half headstand can be done by most people.

Half headstand is how headstand is started. The difference is that you want to get comfortable in half headstand and hold the position without going up into full headstand. Be sure to use plenty of padding, and keep your arms active as described below to keep the pressure off your neck.

Start by kneeling down and place your forearms on the floor in front of you. The ideal distance between your elbows is about forearm length. You can adjust this by holding your elbows with your hands. Then release and move your hands in front where you would interlace your fingers.

Have the arms so the very outer edges of the forearms are on the ground, so the bone is placed on the ground. Specifically, the ulna which is the bone that is on the little finger side of the forearm. Also, have the outside edge of your hand and little finger on the floor.

This triangle is your base. Keep the pressure off your head by activating your arms so this triangle is pressing into the floor when in the pose. Some people can lift their body with this activation, even in full headstand. Avoid lifting completely though, you just want enough activation to keep your neck safe.

Place the crown of your head on the floor with the back of your head cupped in the palms of your hands. There is a tendency to have the hands closed with the palms more together. Keep them open so your palms can wrap around the back of your head.

There is another tendency place closer to the forehead on the floor rather than the crown. Be sure to roll your head further around by moving your chin toward your chest so the very top of your head is on the floor. Ask a friend to check if you're not sure, or consult a yoga instructor.

Next, straighten your legs so your body is in an upside down V shape with your head on one end and toes on the other. Activate your arms as you do this so they are taking most of your weight leaving very little pressure on your head and neck.

From here, walk your feet forward to make your torso more straight up and down. The further you can go (without rolling over) the better.

A slightly deeper diaphragmatic breath is ideal, but not essential for bringing the energy up to the crown chakra. Keep your attention on the crown of your head, generally where it is on the floor, while holding the pose and focusing on the Divine.

Activating the crown chakra brings bliss. This can be the bliss of being whole and total with your relationship with the Divine, or the bliss of having a loving relationship with someone special.

Head Stand -- Crown

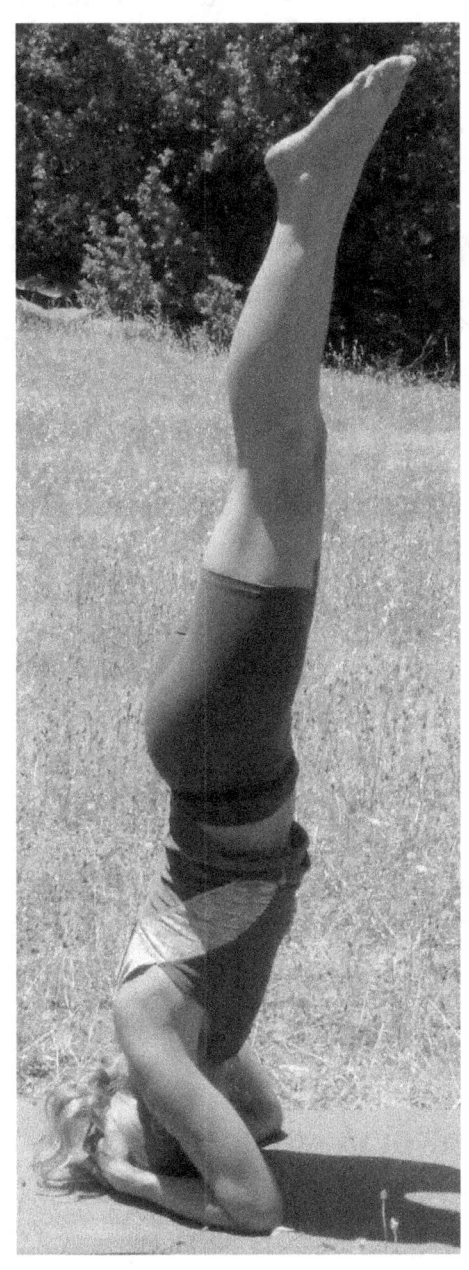

Headstand is the best pose for bringing the energy to the crown chakra. Balance is one of the big difficulties in this pose. You can do it with your back to a wall if you like. Place your hands a few inches away from the wall or you won't be able to stay up.

If balance is particularly difficult you can try doing headstand in a corner so you have two points of contact for your feet to help with balance.

Eventually, you may want to try headstand away from a wall. Make sure there is plenty of room behind you so you can tumble out of the pose if you lose balance. If you go too far and fall over, you can change the fall into a tumble by quickly tucking your chin so you roll out rather than falling and possibly hurting yourself.

Take up the pose by starting in half headstand as described above. Bend your knees and bring your thighs to your body and lift your feet off the floor. Find your balance here without the full extension. Then, slowly lift your legs overhead into the pose.

The ideal position for your feet is together with your toes drawn in rather than pointing. Activate your legs and feet so the soles are reaching strongly up.

It really helps to have a friend spot you until you get the feel for full headstand without a wall. Have them stand so one leg is bent with the inside of their knee and thigh near your back to lightly touching your back so they can easily support you with their leg if you start to fall. They can also hold your ankles as you come up if that helps.

Remember to keep pressing your arms into the floor so you don't compress your neck.

A lot of people practiced headstand as children, usually the tripod headstand with the palms on the floor instead of the forearms. This is much easier for balance, but it is impossible to keep the weight off your head and neck in that position. If you are very sure of yourself, you can try the tripod headstand. I strongly recommend the other version because it is much safer.

To do tripod headstand, start in a similar way as half headstand but with your palms on the floor rather than the forearm method described above. Walk your feet forward and tuck your legs into your body. Make sure your balance is solid in that position before lifting your legs overhead.

Even though you are putting all your weight on your head in this pose, you can still activate your neck muscles lifting your body rather than allowing your neck to relax and compress. Keep this activation throughout the pose.

Keep your attention on the crown chakra as you do your diaphragmatic breathing. Allow your attention to go to the Divine, possibly the non-physical entity that your lover truly is.

The negative emotion associated with the crown chakra is actually a positive. It is called the pain of separation. This pain drives humans to seek union with the Divine. Union with a lover is similar and perhaps the best way to prepare you for union with the formless Divine. Revel in the pain of separation if you find that in your consciousness.

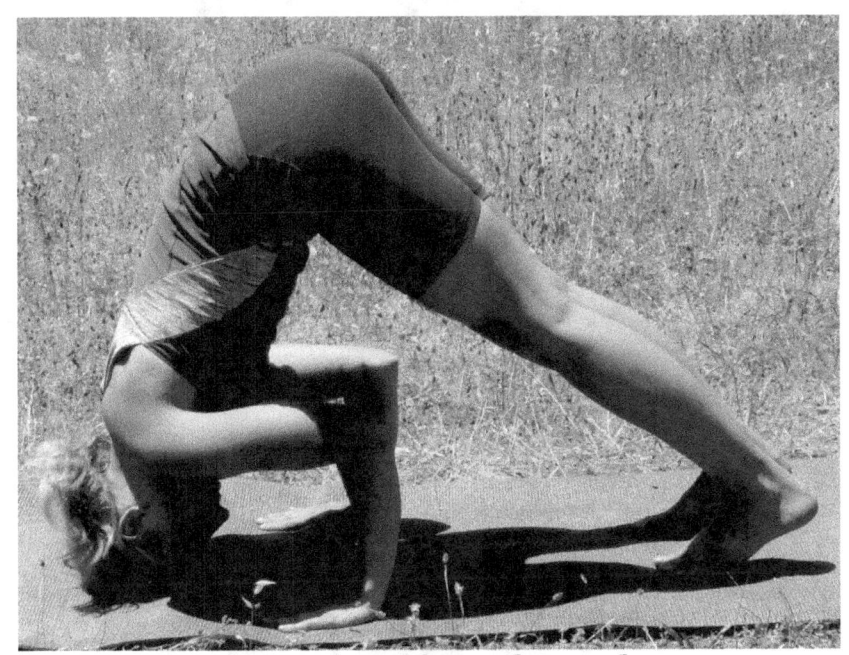

Tripod Half Head Stand

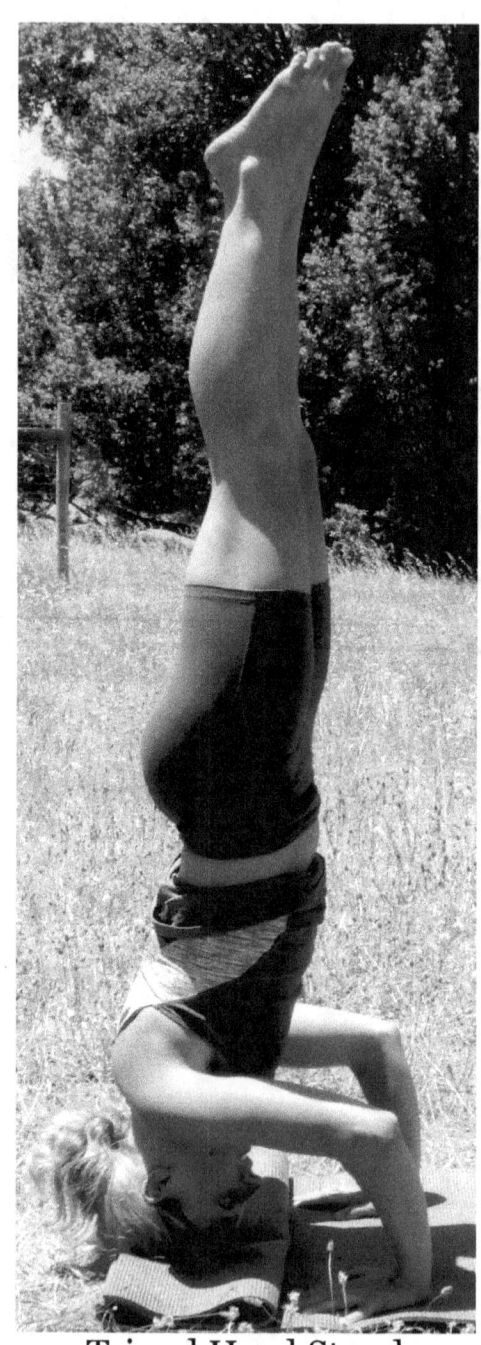

Tripod Head Stand

144

Corpse Pose -- Integration

Corpse pose is done after most yoga classes. Its purpose is to allow the body to relax after a great yoga workout. Another purpose that many yoga instructors may not mention is to integrate the work done.

The main integration done in corpse pose after this class is integrating the energy into both your body and its energy channels. You do this mainly by allowing the energy to flow through your body as you relax.

Feeling the energy in your body and allowing it to flow freely is the main practice for that. The energy knows what is best for you, so be open to having it flow in whatever way is ideal for you.

That means that you will be focusing on two things; relaxing your body, and feeling and allowing the energy flow. Feeling and allowing are counted as the same thing because they are basically surrendering to the energy.

While you are going through the body parts and allowing each to fully relax, keep some attention on the energy in your body as well. You may lose that focus. That's okay, bringing your focus back is a great concentration exercise. And, you can be fully with your energy body when you finish the relaxation meditation.

Corpse pose is usually done while lying on your back. You can modify it for lower back comfort by placing something soft under your knees, as needed.

Alternately, you can relax in child's pose if you like. Or, just lie down on your bed and get comfortable! This is a great way to fall asleep. Whatever works best for you is fine. However, lying on your back is the ideal position for energy flow.

Once you are comfortable lying on your back, place your arms out to the sides far enough away from your body that there is no skin contact in the armpit area.

Rotate your arms back as far as possible, pointing your palms up. Then lift your shoulders slightly and shift your weight on the shoulders so they roll under.

It is usually more comfortable with your shoulders rolled under, and it opens the chest for better energy flow. Relax your arms leaving your palms up.

Spread your legs far enough apart that your feet naturally fall over to the outside when you relax. Adjust your head so that your chin is slightly tucked to take a little of the arch out of the back of your neck. Use a pillow for your head if you like.

Once you are comfortable you can induce a yawn. Yawns are a great relaxation technique themselves. Do this by opening your mouth wide and taking a slow deep inhale through your mouth. Repeat a time or two if you don't get a yawn the first time.

Take time to relax each part of your body as you focus on each individual area. Start by allowing your feet to relax. Let that relaxation up into your calves, then your thighs. Allow your hips and buttocks to relax.

Bring your attention into your torso as you allow your belly to relax. Let organs in your belly relax and release down towards the floor, and into your lower back allowing it to relax.

Bring your attention to your chest and allow it to relax. Take a slightly deeper breath and let it fall out as you fully relax your chest down toward the floor. Allow the relaxation to drain down into your middle back and shoulder blade area.

Next, allow your shoulders to relax and release down into the upper back. Allow your upper arms to relax, the forearms, wrists and hands.

Relax your throat allowing it to open so air flows freely through it, ideally so that you don't hear the inner sound of air passing through as you breathe. Let the relaxation drain into the back of your neck.

Bring your attention into your face and relax your forehead, cheeks, jaw, mouth and tongue. Allow your scalp to relax and drop down toward the floor. Let your head relax with everything draining down so that it feels like the back of your head is sinking into the floor.

Take a minute to scan your body for any area that is tight. As you bring your attention to that area take a deeper breath. Let the breath fall out as you let the area go.

Once you are completely relaxed, bring your attention to the energy in your body. This is a great opportunity to have a good experience of the energy as it flows around your body, especially for anyone without a significant experience of their energy. Allow the energy to flow as it will and simply notice what it does and how it makes you feel.

Most people experience their energy as a feeling. Others may visualize it, while some may get a sense of hearing their energy. Whatever your experience, keep your attention on the energy in your body. Notice what it is doing, where it goes and how it acts.

Keeping your attention on your body's energy can easily bring you to a place where you fall into some form of unconsciousness. Yes, there are different types and levels of unconsciousness and relaxation. You can think of it as sleep though, and allow it if it happens.

As you progress with this class and with yoga in general you may find yourself in deeper and deeper states of relaxation and unconsciousness after a class. Most people will either stay conscious watching their breath and energy, or simply enter something like sleep.

Be sure to set a timer if you need to get up. Or, do this at night and simply have a great sleep!

If you are getting up after corpse pose, come out slowly. Start by slowly wiggling your fingers and toes. Then start to move your hands and feet about. Gradually move your arms and legs around.

Allow yourself to stretch and yawn as you feel. When you are ready, roll onto your right side and lie there for a moment before pushing yourself up to a sitting position.

Take another few moments to notice how you feel and what is going on with your body, energy, state of mind etc. before getting on with the rest of your day.

Bringing it Together

You now have all the pieces for you to accomplish the ultimate ejaculation restraint! Let's put it all together with a review and some practical practice.

During sex you will have different experiences with your restraint depending on where you are in your practice of the techniques taught in this book.

At first you may just stop yourself from orgasm and ejaculation when you first start to feel orgasm coming on. This is the first level of restraint which will be a great accomplishment for many men.

When you start to feel an orgasm coming on you withdraw, stop for a minute and squeeze the PC muscle while the orgasmic energy passes, probably by holding for a minute or so. It could take much less time for some men, perhaps longer for others. It is completely individual.

The main point is that you will be able to quickly go back to having sex for a much longer session of intercourse for you and your partner's prolonged pleasure.

That is a major accomplishment which will make you one of the best lovers your partner is likely to have. You will be able to choose whether or not to have an orgasm and ejaculation as you wish.

Orgasm can take a few seconds to actually happen. So, a deeper level of ability is to move into the orgasm somewhat. That is the second level of restraint; to be able to experience moving into the orgasm somewhat and still be able to restrain before it gets really intense.

That may require a little more strength in both the PC muscle as well as in the general health and strength of your body. The three locks may even occur at this level. At the very least you would want to work with inducing the locks so your ability can become even greater.

The third level of ability is to have a full internal orgasm without ejaculating. That can happen with or without the breath of fire.

But, at that level you really should start working with the breath of fire to keep increasing your ability, and to insure that you can restrain completely.

These three levels could be broken up even more, but that is the basic idea of how things will progress. Keep practicing and working with yourself and with your partner during lovemaking to continue increasing in ability.

Practices

These practices put together all the parts the way they would happen at the deepest level of restraint. It would be best if you first had a good experience of the locks, and were able to do the breath of fire reasonably well.

The first exercise is to put the pieces together while sitting in half or full lotus. You might also try just sitting comfortably cross legged, or even in a chair since that is a position you could be in during sex. Sitting cross legged is particularly good for anyone interested in learning advanced red tantra techniques.

While sitting comfortably, do a round of breath of fire. Instead of inhaling and holding your breath you will simply very quickly at the end of your 30 or so quick breaths. Hold the exhale as you induce or let happen the three locks. If you're not getting the locks yet, simply squeeze your PC muscle as hard as you can.

While squeezing the PC muscle is how you induce the root lock, it is also your primary restraint technique, so you want to have that going as strongly as possible.

Inhale when you need to, but keep squeezing your PC muscle. Try to keep the PC squeezing at least a total of one minute.

Work up to increasing the squeeze time to about two minutes with this exercise since that is the longest you are likely to need to hold to restrain an ejaculation. Actually, the longest will usually be less than a minute, but it is best to train for more.

Next, try the same practice but while in serpent pose to simulate having sex in the missionary position (face to face with the man on top). You can push up on you knees slightly to make the position more realistic.

The next exercise is to actually restrain an ejaculation with all the pieces put together as above. The only difference is that you will only do the breath of fire contractions until you need to exhale to hold the breath. You would start breath of fire as your orgasm starts to come on, and exhale completely when you squeeze the PC muscle.

You can do this in whatever position you masturbate in, probably lying on your back if you're like most men. Lying face down or on your side are other common positions, they will all work for this practice.

The last exercise is to put all the parts together while masturbating in a sitting position. A lot of men may find this difficult to impossible, but give it a try. If needed, you can sit up when you get close to orgasm.

As you practice you will be getting the timing of when to start the breath of fire and when to very quickly exhale all the air for holding the exhale. This may take time to figure out. You will likely continue to refine your technique as you become a better lover.

Doing this practice whenever you masturbate is ideal. If you get to that place where you just have to have an ejaculation then do the practice anyway, you can always chose to let go at most any time, even if you have started restraining.

Becoming Multiply Orgasmic

Once you master these techniques you will likely become multiply orgasmic. This is an amazing place to be in, especially if you have a compatible partner.

This is the ultimate internal orgasm. That is, an orgasm that happens inside your body rather than having the outward experience that comes with an ejaculation.

This is close to what multiply orgasmic women experience. The ease with which women can have an orgasm move up their spine is why they are so often multiply orgasmic. Sharing that with a loving partner is truly an amazing experience.

If you are with a very compatible partner she will most likely orgasm with you each time. If she isn't completely compatible with you in that way she may get there with you as your ability increases.

Of course, you may need to help her to become multiply orgasmic. The details of that are for another book, but having long sex sessions is one of the ways.

One partner I had and I would have at least 50 orgasms in a long sex session. I could never count them all, but at times it surely exceeded 100. At times like those we would have sexual intercourse for three to five hours. Total time making love could easily reach eight hours or more! I still can't figure out why she broke up with me!!

An interesting point is that without the satisfaction of an ejaculation you will want to and be able to continue having intercourse for long periods of time. All the while not satisfied! That is a frustrating place to be in, often *very* frustrating.

This brings up another ability that has to be developed; being able to deny yourself that ultimate satisfaction for your partner's greater satisfaction.

For me, the act of intercourse has become satisfying in a different way. First, the sensation of the penis in the vagina has become generally preferable to having an orgasm. And, seeing my partner in the throes of orgasm again and again is a different kind of indescribable satisfaction.

At some point though, there needs to be a stopping point. Usually, an ejaculation has to occur or frustration is all that you will be left with once you stop. A single drop of ejaculate can be enough though. I call it "the drop that satisfies."

Getting to the place where you can deny yourself that final satisfaction is another level that starts to become spiritual. It is not that common, but some men may find themselves there. They are the ones who may want to know even more about the deeper aspects of this practice.

One issue you are likely to encounter is that you might want to continue having intercourse while your partner might need you to stop. She may not have the same capacity as you.

For one thing, her skin may be more sensitive than yours. Remember, you have been practicing with masturbation which may have toughened your skin. You may have to accommodate her until she toughens up!

Another thing that can happen is that she may not be able to tolerate that much pleasure! You may literally fuck her brains out! It's an amazing experience to see your lover give up and go beyond anything she's ever experienced before. The look of total surrender on her face can be amazing to witness!

Whichever case, if she won't let you continue as long as you want, you may have to take a break. More likely though, you will need to have her tell you when she is a few minutes away from not being able to take anymore so you can let yourself ejaculate. Or, you might try just letting that drop that satisfies escape.

Always remember, if you make pleasing your partner more important than your needs then you **will** be a better lover!

Conclusion

Gaining the ability to restrain your ejaculation is something that just about everyone should be able to do. The only limit might be some physical or medical condition. Now that you have the secrets to developing this high ability, you too should find yourself able to surprise your lover(s).

An important part of it is to notice the timing of things. Like, when you start out you may need to do the technique of having sex before sex. How long before getting together with your partner is ideal? Too long and you may be too sensitive again, too soon and not sensitive enough.

Timing is also important in knowing when to stop and hold to keep from having an orgasm. As your timing gets better, and you start to notice the separation between orgasm and ejaculation, you may be able to have an orgasm without ejaculating and be able to easily continue lovemaking after restraining.

The most important thing you have to do is to develop your PC muscle's strength. The great thing about that is that you can do it pretty much anywhere and anytime! That will bring you results faster than anything else.

If you continue with what is recommended in this book you are very likely to become multiply orgasmic. While that will be really great for you, your climax will likely bring her to orgasm as well, if she is a very compatible lover. The energy that develops in your body from these practices can greatly influence what happens to her. And, she will absolutely love it!!

As you grow and develop your abilities, you will start to increase in other lovemaking abilities like keeping your attention on her, knowing what she wants and needs by where her attention goes, your new sensitivity will even be reflected in how you touch her, and your touch may become more electrifying to her.

Learning to make love in the way taught in this book will very likely make your life with your lover a great adventure with amazing experiences for both of you. That is my wish for you both!

About the Author

Kalidasa is currently based in the Russian River area of Northern California. He is a long time yoga instructor, holistic healer and tantra practitioner. He has worked with individuals and groups for over 30 years.

His strong desire to help people learn to help themselves has led him to writing books on health, yoga and tantric techniques. His current books are listed below.

He has spent his life meditating, teaching yoga and developing unique techniques that that have impacted thousands of people. He has recently come out of seclusion to offer more information for the benefit of others.

He is the developer of Self Adjusting Technique (SAT), a method of doing gentle adjustments on yourself so chiropractic adjustments can be avoided. The simple adjustments don't require force or cracking, so they are much more appealing to people who don't like that type of work. You can learn about SAT and other healing techniques as well as what his healing private sessions are by visiting http://selfadjustingtechnique.com

His new site, http://kalidasa.com has more information about Kalidasa and some of the practices mentioned in this book.

You can contact him through either site about private or group sessions.

Books by Kalidasa

Self Adjusting Technique

Teaches you how to do adjustments on yourself so you can avoid visits to the chiropractor. The adjustments are very gentle with no force or cracking involved.

The adjustments are based on the principle that your body goes in and out of alignment all the time. The body simply adjusts itself by means of muscles pulling on the bones combined with movement to easily slip joints back into proper alignment.

Tight muscles prevent this natural realignment, but you can do the same thing with gentle pressure and easy movements to realign yourself naturally.

Included are adjustment techniques for the neck, back, hips and ribs.

Adrenal Fatigue: Get Your Life Back

Adre3nal fatigue is the hidden condition that most doctors know little to nothing about. Multiple symptoms and conditions completely baffle most doctors who just throw medications at the problems to see what might help. Now you can truly take your life back by understanding this little known but all too common condition.

Eliminate Fat Hormones for Weight Loss and Health -Lose Weight and Prevent Cancer with Supplements

Estrogenic cancer is the most deadly type of cancer. It is caused by the liver not making the hormone water soluble for elimination. Estrogen is also the fat hormone that makes fat deposit in the body. Giving the liver the nutrients needed to eliminate estrogen both prevents cancer, and aids in weight loss.

Yoga for Lower Back Pain

This is an easy to follow yoga class with poses that are of great help to most back pain issues. Plenty of information on how to care for your back is included.

Yoga for the Psoas

The deepest muscle in the body is the same one that Pilates is designed to strengthen. The psoas muscle is easy to stretch if you now the right techniques. Over 40 different stretches and variations to give your psoas the best stretch it can have.

Floor Yoga Class

A simple yet complete yoga class that is done completely on the floor. Perfect for the beginner or limited yoga practitioner.